AF477200

Career Opportunities in Pharmacy

Career Opportunities in Pharmacy

D K Tripathi

Professor & Principal

Rungta College of Pharmaceutical Sciences & Research,
Bhilai.

and

Ex - Dean & Chairman

BoS Pharmacy,
Chhattisgarh Swami Vivekanand Technical University
Bhilai.

P K Sahu

Professor
School of Pharmaceutical Sciences
(SPS).
Siksha O Anusandhan University,
Kalinga Nagar, Ghatikia,
Bhubaneswar

T R Satpathy

Placement Co-ordinator
School of Pharmaceutical Sciences
(SPS).
Siksha O Anusandhan University,
Kalinga Nagar, Ghatikia,
Bhubaneswar

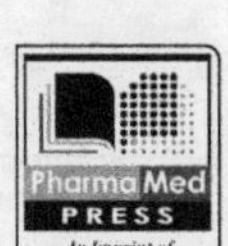

PharmaMed Press

An imprint of Pharma Book Syndicate

A unit of BSP Books Pvt. Ltd.

4-4-309/316, Giriraj Lane,
Sultan Bazar, Hyderabad - 500 095.

Career Opportunities in Pharmacy *by D K Tripathi, P K Sahu and T R Satpathy*

© 2019, *by Publisher,* All rights reserved.

No part of this book or parts thereof may be reproduced, stored in a retrieval system or transmitted in any language or by any means, electronic, mechanical, photocopying, recording or otherwise without the prior written permission of the publishers.

Published by

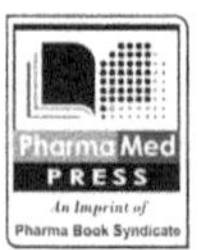

PharmaMed Press

An imprint of Pharma Book Syndicate

A unit of BSP Books Pvt. Ltd.
4-4-309/316, Giriraj Lane, Sultan Bazar, Hyderabad - 500 095.
Phone: 040-23445688, 23445600; Fax: 91+40-23445611
E-mail: info@pharmamedpress.com
www.pharmamedpress.com/pharmamedpress.net

ISBN: 978-93-88305-00-6 (Hardback)

PREFACE

The students who are admitted to Pharmacy course irrespective of level do not know what they can do after completion. Moreover the people of our country are not fully aware of the future options. Just as a technical course they put their wards with an understanding that at least a medical shop can be opened and run to maintain livelihood or their sons will get a job of medical representative.

In fact, many students choose this course out of compulsion, not as a first choice (passion). This is due to lack of awareness about the prospect of this course among common people. Moreover, the students are not being informed by their mentors of what the options are after completion of the course.

Hence, a gap has been existing between what can be done and what is being done and someone at some point of time has to bridge the gap. It is of immense pleasure that our colleague Dr. Pratap Kumar Sahu working in SOA University, Bhubaneswar, Odisha as Professor took the pain to gather and compile all the relevant information related to career opportunity in Pharmacy. This ultimately resulted the book named **Career Opportunities in Pharmacy.**

We strongly believe that the book would definitely help the students to select future options after completion of the course in Pharmacy. Besides, the students who are pursuing school education if read the book would know the career options in Pharmacy.

- Authors

CONTENTS

Preface .... (v)

CHAPTER 1

What is Pharmacy? 1

CHAPTER 2

History of Pharmacy 3

CHAPTER 3

Courses in Pharmacy 5

CHAPTER 4

Career Opportunities in Pharmacy

    4.1 Pharmaceutical Industry 14

    4.2 Pharmaceutical Marketing 21

    4.3 Drug Administration (State & Central)......... 28

    4.4 Entrepreneurship 32

    4.5 Academics 32

    4.6 Clinical Research 32

    4.7 Hospital (Govt. & Private) 38

    4.8 IT & Insurance... 45

    4.9 Miscellaneous 51

CHAPTER 5

Interview

5.1 Introduction 59

5.2 Task to do before Attending the Interview 62

5.3 Questions Most Frequently Asked by HR /
     Other Experts About You 63

5.4 Questions Asked by Different Experts of
     Pharma Industry 67

5.5 Questions for Medical Representatives 88

5.6 Questions for Hospital & Retail Pharmacy 93

5.7 Questions for Pharmacovigilance &
     Clinical Data Management (CDM) 94

CHAPTER 6

Few Employers 111

APPENDIX

List of Few Pharmaceutical Industries 119

CHAPTER 1

What is Pharmacy?

Pharmacy is the science and technique of preparing and dispensing drugs and medicines. It is a health profession that links the health sciences with the chemical sciences and aims to ensure the safe and effective use of pharmaceuticals or drugs.

The Greek word pharmakon means "drug" or "medicine".

Pharmacists, therefore, are the experts of drugs who not only manufacture medicines but also optimize use of medication for the benefit of the patients.

Pharmacy can be defined in the following ways:

- It is the science of medicinal substances comprising of Pharmacology, Phytochemistry, Pharmacognosy, Pharmaceutics, and Pharmaceutical chemistry.
- It is a place where prescription medicines are dispensed.
- The occupation of Pharmacist is known as Pharmacy.
- It is also considered as the art of preparing medicinal products, or a place where such substances are sold.
- It is the study of the preparation and dispensing of medications.
- It is the branch of health sciences dealing with the preparation, storage and proper utilization of medicinal products.

So, Pharmacy is a health profession which is concerned with the design, production, evaluation and proper / rational use of medicine. It links the health science with the biological, chemical and medical science.

A **Pharmacist** is a person whose profession is Pharmacy. In India the minimum qualification for registration as a Pharmacist is "Diploma course in Pharmacy" (D.Pharm) or "Degree course in Pharmacy" (B.Pharm) or "Doctor of Pharmacy" (Pharm D) from an institution approved u/s 12 of the Pharmacy Act, 1948.

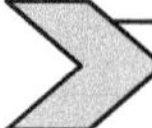

Pharmaceutical Associations

A Pharmacist can be a member of following associations:

- The International Pharmaceutical Federation (**FIP**)
  www.fip.org
- Indian Pharmaceutical Association (**IPA**)
  www.ipapharma.org
- Indian Pharmaceutical Congress Association (**IPCA**)
  www.scientificipca.org

Indian Pharmaceutical Congress Association (IPCA) is the apex body representing the Pharmaceutical working in various disciplines and areas of work. It is a federation of 5 National Pharmaceutical Associations as its constituents which includes

1. Indian Pharmaceutical Association (**IPA**)

   www.ipapharma.org

2. Indian Pharmacy Graduate's Association (**IPGA**)

   www.ipga.in

3. Indian Hospitals Pharmacists Association (**IHPA**)

   www.ihpa.co.in

4. The Association of Pharma Teachers of India (**APTI**)

   www.aptiindia.org

5. The All India Drugs Control Officers Confederation (**AIDCOC**)

   www.aidcoc.in

CHAPTER 2

History of Pharmacy

Evolution of Pharmacy, Pharmacists and Pharmacopoeias has taken place differently in different countries across the World based on the prevailing socio-economic and educational background. Few examples are given below:

- Many Sumerian (late 6000-2000 BC) cuneiform clay tablets record prescriptions for medicine.

- Ancient Egyptian pharmacological knowledge was recorded in various papyri such as the Ebers Papyrus of 1550BC, and the Edwin Smith Papyrus of the 16th century BC.

- The Greek physician Pedanius Dioscorides is famous for writing a five volume book in his native Greek in the 1st century AD. The Latin translation De Materia Medica (Concerning medical substances) was used as a basis for many medieval texts.

- The earliest known Chinese manual on materia medica is the Shennong Bencao Jing (The Divine Farmer's Herb-Root Classic), dating back to the 100AD.

- In Japan, at the end of the Asuka period (538-710 AD) and the early Nara period (710-794 AD), the men who fulfilled roles similar to those of modern pharmacists were highly respected. The place of pharmacists in the society was specifically defined in the Taiho Code (701 AD) and re-stated in the Yoro Code (718 AD).

- There is a stone sign for a pharmacy with a tripod, a mortar, and a pestle opposite one for a doctor in the Arcadian Way in Ephesus near Kusadasi in Turkey. The current Ephesus dates back to 400 BC.

- In Baghdad the first pharmacies, or drug stores, were established in 754, under the Abbasid Caliphate during the Islamic Golden Age. By the 9th century, these pharmacies were state-regulated.

- The advances made in the Middle East in botany and chemistry led medicine in medieval Islam substantially to develop pharmacology. Muhammad ibn Zakariya Razi (Rhazes) (865-915 CE), for instance, acted to promote the medical uses of chemical compounds. Abu al-Qasim al-Zahrawi (Abulcasis) (936-1013CE) pioneered the preparation of medicines by sublimation and distillation. Sabur Ibn Sahl (869 CE), was, however, the first physician to initiate pharmacopoedia, describing a large variety of drugs and remedies for ailments. Al-Biruni (973-1050 AD) wrote one of the most valuable Islamic works on pharmacology entitled Kitab al-Saydalah (The Book of Drugs), where he gave detailed knowledge of the properties of drugs and outlined the role of pharmacy and the functions and duties of the pharmacist. Avicenna, too, described no less than 700 preparations, their properties, mode of action and their indications.

- In Europe pharmacy-like shops began to appear during the 12th century. In 1240 emperor Frederic II issued a decree by which the physician's and the apothecary's professions were separated. The first pharmacy in Europe (still working) was opened in 1241 in Trier, Germany.

- The Sushruta Samhita is known as the earliest compilation of medicinal substances in India. It is an Indian Ayurvedic treatise since 6th century BC. The Pharmacy Council of India is the statutory body of government of India also called as central council constituted under the Pharmacy Act, 1948. The Council was first constituted on 4 March 1948. The Drugs and Cosmetics Act, 1940 is an Act of the Parliament of India which regulates the import, manufacture, distribution and sale of drugs in India. The Drugs and Cosmetics Rules, 1945 are the set of rules under The Drugs and Cosmetics Act, 1940 which contains provisions for classification of drugs under given schedules and there are guidelines for the storage, sale, display and prescription of each schedule.

- A pharmacopoeia is a book containing directions for the identification of compound, medicines and published by the authority of a government or a medical or pharmaceutical society. The term Pharmacopoeia first appears as a distinct title in a work published at Basel, Switzerland, in 1561 by A. Foes but does not appear to have come into general use until the beginning of the 17th century. Few Pharmacopeias published in 17th century were Pharmacopoeia of Amsterdam (Pharmacopoea Amstelredamensis) in 1636, London Pharmacopoeia in 1618, Edinburgh Pharmacopoeia in 1699 and Dublin Pharmacopoeia in 1807. The Medical Act of 1858 ordained that the General Medical Council should publish a book containing a list of medicines and compounds, to be called the British Pharmacopoeia, which would be a substitute throughout Great Britain and Ireland for the separate Pharmacopoeias. Similarly many national and international Pharmacopoeias, like the EU and the U.S. Pharmacopoeias were published 19th century onwards. In India, the actual process of publishing the first Pharmacopoeia started in the year 1944 under the chairmanship of Col. R. N. Chopra. The first edition of Indian Pharmacopeia was published in the year 1955 and the 8th edition of Indian Pharmacopeia is published in the year 2018.

CHAPTER 3

Courses in Pharmacy

D.Pharm is a two years course after 10+2 (science academic stream) followed by 500 hours of practical training spread over a period of 3 months. B.Pharm is a 4 years course after 10+2 (science stream). Pharm D is a 6 years (5+1) course after 10+2 (science stream). D. Pharm and Pharm D courses are clinical oriented whereas B. Pharm course is industry oriented. One can pursue M. Pharm after B. Pharm in different specializations. *Pharm. D. (Post Baccalaureate)* is a 3-year professional post-graduate course in the discipline of Pharmacy, open for pursuance by eligible graduates of Pharmacy.

Name of the Course	Duration	Eligibility
D. Pharm	2 years & 3 months	10+2 Science
B. Pharm	4 years	10+2 Science
B. Pharmacy Practice	2 years	D. Pharm and A minimum of four years of pharmacy practice experience in a community or hospital pharmacy
Pharm. D	**6 years including 1 year internship**	10+2 Science
	3 years including 1 year internship	B.Pharm
M.Pharm	2 years	B.Pharm
MBA	2 years	B.Pharm
PG Diploma	1 year	B.Pharm
Ph. D.	3-7 years	M.Pharm/Pharm.D

- **D. Pharm (Diploma in Pharmacy)**

  Basically diploma is conducted on board level. Pharmacy Council of India (PCI) has established a uniform and unique syllabus for all the colleges in different states across India.

Total Subjects to study.

Part-I

Subject	No. of hours of Theory	No. of hours Practical
Pharmaceutics-I	75	100
Pharmaceutical Chemistry-I	75	75
Pharmacognosy	75	75
Biochemistry and Clinical Pathology	50	75
Human Anatomy and Physiology	75	50
Health Education and Community Pharmacy	50	-
Total	400	375=775

Part-II

Subject	No. of hours of Theory	No. of hours of Practical
Pharmaceutics-II	75	100
Pharmaceutical Chemistry-II	100	75
Pharmacology and Toxicology	75	50
Pharmaceutical Jurisprudence	50	-
Drug Store and Business Management	75	-
Hospital and Clinical pharmacy	75	50
Total	450	275=725

Duration:

2 years plus practical training of 500 hours spread over a period of not less than 3 months in Govt. Hospital/Pharmacy, recognized by Pharmacy Council of India, New Delhi.

- **B. Pharm (Bachelor of Pharmacy)**

B.Pharm is a graduation course in Pharmacy. One can pursue this course in India after pre university studies or 12th standard in Science and it requires 4 years of college studies. To take admission in B.Pharm one should have Physics, Chemistry with Biology or Mathematics or Biotechnology or Computer Science as his/her +2 Science subjects. Students from Diploma in Pharmacy can directly enter into 2nd year of B.Pharm (Lateral entry).

Pharmacy Council of India (PCI) has established a unique syllabus for all the colleges in different states.

Semester I: Human Anatomy and Physiology I, Pharmaceutical Analysis I, Pharmaceutics I, Pharmaceutical Inorganic Chemistry, Communication skills, Remedial Biology / Remedial Mathematics.

Semester II: Human Anatomy and Physiology II, Pharmaceutical Organic Chemistry I, Biochemistry, Pathophysiology, Computer Applications in Pharmacy, Environmental sciences

Semester III: Pharmaceutical Organic Chemistry II, Physical Pharmaceutics I, Pharmaceutical Microbiology, Pharmaceutical Engineering

Semester IV: Pharmaceutical Organic Chemistry III, Medicinal Chemistry I, Physical Pharmaceutics II, Pharmacology I, Pharmacognosy and Phytochemistry I.

Semester V: Medicinal Chemistry II, Industrial Pharmacy I, Pharmacology II, Pharmacognosy and Phytochemistry II, Pharmaceutical Jurisprudence.

Semester VI: Medicinal Chemistry III, Pharmacology III, Herbal Drug Technology, Biopharmaceutics and Pharmacokinetics, Pharmaceutical Biotechnology, Quality Assurance.

Semester VII: Instrumental Methods of Analysis, Industrial Pharmacy II, Pharmacy Practice, Novel Drug Delivery System.

Semester VIII: Biostatistics and Research Methodology, Social and Preventive Pharmacy, Pharma Marketing Management, Pharmaceutical Regulatory Science, Pharmacovigilance, Quality Control and Standardization of Herbals, Computer Aided Drug Design, Cell and Molecular Biology, Cosmetic Science, Experimental Pharmacology, Advanced Instrumentation Techniques, Dietary Supplements and Nutraceuticals, Project Work.

- **Bachelor of Pharmacy Practice (Bridge course)**

Bachelor of Pharmacy Practice - It consists of a degree certificate of having passed the course of study and examination as prescribed in these regulations, for the purpose of additional qualification to be entered in Register of Pharmacist under the Pharmacy Act, 1948. The duration of the course shall be of two academic years with each year spread over a period of not less than 180 working days.

Minimum qualification for admission to the course is:

- A Diploma holder in Pharmacy Course from an institution approved by Pharmacy Council of India approved under section 12 of the Pharmacy Act 1948.
- A Minimum of four years of pharmacy practice experience in a community or hospital pharmacy.

According to Pharmacy Council of India (PCI) the syllabus is as follows:

1st Year: Pathophysiology and Pharmacotherapeutics I, Pathophysiology and Pharmacotherapeutics II, Pharmacy Practice I, Pharmacy Practice II, Applied Pharmaceutics, Social Pharmacy I.

2nd Year: Pathophysiology and Pharmacotherapeutics III, Pathophysiology and Pharmacotherapeutics IV, Pharmacy Practice III, Pharmacy Practice IV, Social Pharmacy II, Pharmaceutical Jurisprudence.

- **Pharm. D (Doctor of Pharmacy)**

  Pharm. D is a 6 years course including 1 year internship. One can pursue Pharm. D after +2 Science. B.Pharm graduate is needed to study only 2 years and 1 year of hospital training to complete Doctor of Pharmacy.

  The basic objective of Pharm D is to produce trained manpower for

  - Collaborating with other healthcare professionals for safe and effective pharmaceutical care,
  - Disease management,
  - Pharmaco economics (Effective & cost efficient care),
  - Tracking Adverse Drug Reaction (ADR),
  - Patient Counseling,
  - Monitoring patient outcome etc.

- **M.Pharm (Master of Pharmacy)**

  One can pursue this course in India after B. Pharm only and it requires 2 years of college studies.

  There are number of specializations in M.Pharm like Pharmaceutics, Industrial Pharmacy, Pharmaceutical Chemistry, Pharmaceutical Analysis, Pharmaceutical Quality Assurance, Pharmaceutical Regulatory Affairs, Pharmaceutical Biotechnology, Pharmacy Practice, Pharmacology, Pharmacognosy.

I year: (Semester I & Semester II)

PHARMACEUTICS:

Semester I: Modern Analytical Techniques, Drug Delivery System (DDS), Modern Pharmaceutics, Regulatory Affair.

Semester II: Molecular Pharmaceutics (Nano Tech and Targeted DDS), Advanced Biopharmaceutics & Pharmacokinetics, Computer Aided Drug Delivery System, Cosmetic and Cosmeceuticals.

INDUSTRIAL PHARMACY:

Semester I: Modern Pharmaceutical Analytical Techniques, Pharmaceutical Formulation Development, Novel drug delivery systems, Intellectual Property Rights.

Semester II: Advanced Biopharmaceutics and Pharmacokinetics, Scale up and Technology Transfer, Pharmaceutical Production Technology, Entrepreneurship Management.

PHARMACEUTICAL CHEMISTRY:

Semester I: Modern Pharmaceutical Analytical Techniques, Advanced Organic Chemistry–I, Advanced Medicinal Chemistry, Chemistry of Natural Products.

Semester II: Advanced Spectral Analysis, Advanced Organic Chemistry–II, Computer Aided Drug Design, Pharmaceutical Process Chemistry.

PHARMACEUTICAL ANALYSIS:

Semester I: Modern Pharmaceutical Analytical Techniques Advanced Pharmaceutical Analysis, Pharmaceutical Validation, Food Analysis.

Semester II: Advanced Instrumental Analysis, Modern Bio-Analytical Techniques, Quality Control and Quality Assurance, Herbal and Cosmetic Analysis.

PHARMACEUTICAL QUALITY ASSURANCE:

Semester I: Modern Pharmaceutical Analytical Techniques, Quality Management System, Quality Control and Quality Assurance, Product Development and Technology Transfer.

Semester II: Hazards and Safety Management, Pharmaceutical Validation, Audits and Regulatory Compliance, Pharmaceutical Manufacturing Technology.

REGULATORY AFFAIRS:

Semester I: Good Regulatory Practices, Documentation and Regulatory Writing, Clinical Research Regulations, Regulations and Legislation for Drugs & Cosmetics, Medical Devices, Biologicals & Herbals, and Food & Nutraceuticals in India and Intellectual Property Rights.

Semester II: Regulatory Aspects of Drugs & Cosmetics, Regulatory Aspects of Herbal & Biologicals, Regulatory Aspects of Medical Devices, Regulatory Aspects of Food & Nutraceuticals.

PHARMACEUTICAL BIOTECHNOLOGY:

Semester I: Modern Pharmaceutical Analytical Techniques, Microbial and Cellular Biology, Bioprocess Engineering and Technology, Advanced Pharmaceutical Biotechnology.

Semester II: Proteins and protein Formulation, Immunotechnology, Bioinformatics and Computer Technology, Biological Evaluation of Drug Therapy.

PHARMACY PRACTICE:

Semester I: Clinical Pharmacy Practice, Pharmacotherapeutics-I, Hospital & Community Pharmacy, Clinical Research, Principles of Quality Use of Medicines.

Semester II: Principles of Quality Use of Medicines, Pharmacotherapeutics II, Clinical Pharmacokinetics and Therapeutic Drug Monitoring, Pharmacoepidemiology & Pharmacoeconomics.

PHARMACOLOGY:

Semester I: Modern Pharmaceutical Analytical Techniques, Advanced Pharmacology-I, Pharmacological and Toxicological Screening Methods-I, Cellular and Molecular Pharmacology.

Semester II: Advanced Pharmacology II, Pharmacological and Toxicological Screening Methods-II, Principles of Drug Discovery.

PHARMACOGNOSY:

Semester I: Modern Pharmaceutical Analytical Techniques, Advanced Pharmacognosy-1, Phytochemistry, Industrial Pharmacognostical Technology.

Semester II: Medicinal Plant Biotechnology, Advanced Pharmacognosy-II, Indian System of Medicine, Herbal cosmetics.

II year: (Semester III & Semester IV)

Semester III: (Common for all Specializations): Research Methodology and Biostatistics, Journal club, Discussion / Presentation (Proposal Presentation), Research Work.

Semester IV: Journal Club, Research Work.

- **M.B.A**

Master studies in Business Administration (MBA). One can pursue this course after B.Pharm. And it requires 2 years of college studies. One can pursue MBA in distance mode also. In addition to regular MBA specialization one can pursue MBA (Pharma) also.

- **PG Diploma Courses**

  Now as per recent market needs there are so many PG diploma courses available. This includes clinical research, drug regulatory affairs, Intellectual Property Rights, Pharmacovigilance, Clinical Data Management, SAP and SAS etc. These all are either part time courses or full time courses.

- **Ph.D.**

  One can pursue Ph.D. (Doctor of Philosophy) in Pharmacy from different Universities after M.Pharm.

CHAPTER 4

Career Opportunities in Pharmacy

There are many career opportunities for Pharmacists after D.Pharm/ B.Pharm/ M.Pharm/ Pharm. D (Figure 4.1).

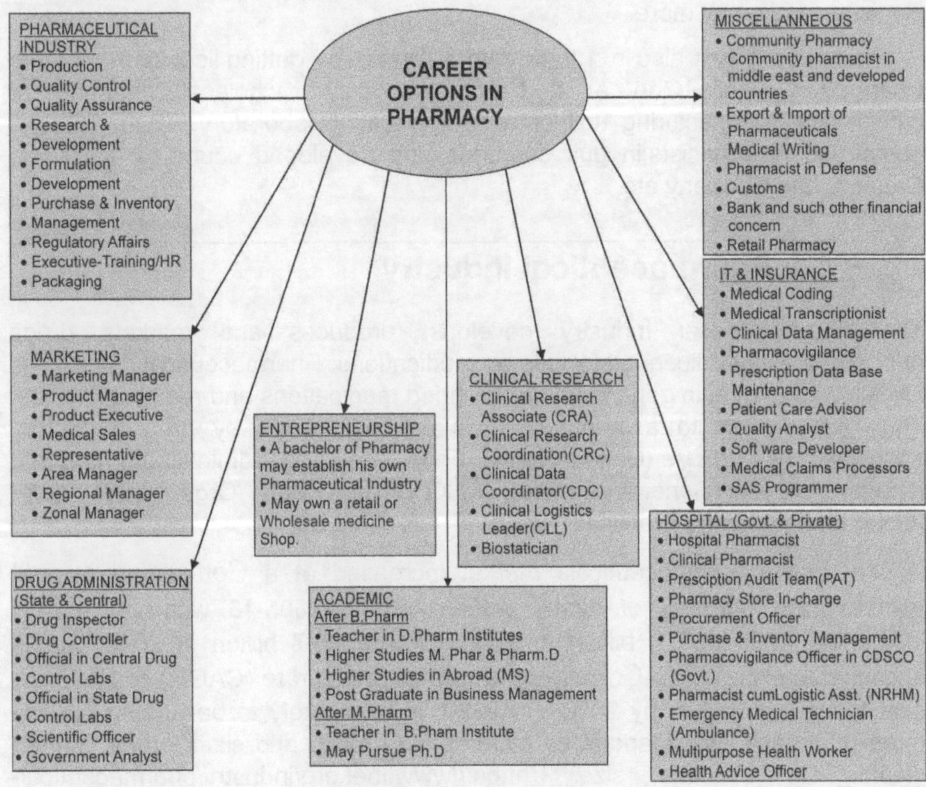

Fig. 4.1 Career Options in Pharmacy.

D.Pharm and Pharm D students can directly join Hospitals, Clinics, and Nursing Homes etc. where as B.Pharm and M.Pharm can join in Sales, Production, Research and Development (R&D), Formulation and Development (F&D), Quality Assurance (QA), Quality Control (QC), Clinical Research (CR), Drug Regulatory Affairs (DRA), Intellectual Property Rights (IPR), Pharmacovigilance (PV), Medical Coding, Hospitals and also in IT firms. Pharm D people can also join in Clinical Research, Pharmacovigilance and Medical Coding etc.

A lot of jobs are available in Pharmaceutical industry. Many times getting jobs is tough as it requires some recommendation. The other reasons is that many companies are associated with placement agencies, soo one may not get a job without referring from placement agency. Only it requires a proper channel to go through with adequate preparation.

Government sectors are booming for pharmacist in different areas like Faculty jobs (Teaching), Hospital Pharmacy, Drug Inspectors, Govt. Analyst, Registrar and many more.

Pharmacists can also run their own business by getting license from State Pharmacy Councils. One can start retail pharmacy or wholesale pharmacy or can own a manufacturing unit or a quality testing laboratory. There is huge demand of Pharmacists in gulf countries and developed countries like USA, Canada, and Germany etc.

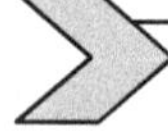

4.1 Pharmaceutical Industry

The Pharmaceutical Industry develops, produces and markets drugs or pharmaceuticals licensed for use as medications. Pharmaceutical companies are allowed to deal in generic and/or branded medications and medical devices. They are subject to a variety of laws and regulations by drug regulatory agencies like USFDA (United States Food and drug administration), DCGI (Drugs Controller General of India), WHO (World Health Organization) GMP (Good Manufacturing Practices) etc.

The Indian pharmaceuticals market increased at a Compound annual growth rate (CAGR) of 17.46 percent during 2005-16 with the market increasing from US$ 6 billion in 2005 to US$ 36.7 billion in 2016 and is expected to expand at a Compound annual growth rate (CAGR) of 15.92 per cent to US$ 55 billion by 2020. By 2020, India is likely to be among the top three pharmaceutical markets by incremental growth and sixth largest market globally in absolute size. (https://www.ibef.org/industry/pharmaceutical-india.aspx)

World wide, Indian drugs are exported to more than 200 countries, including US as the key market. On the global front, the IPM is ranked 13th in terms of value. Owing to robust growth, its ranking is expected to improve to 11th position by 2018. (https:// www.equitymaster.com/research-it/sector-info/ pharma/Pharmaceuticals-Sector-Analysis-Report.asp)

An extensive list of Pharmaceutical Industries is given in Appendix 1.

The Pharmaceutical Industries have the following departments

4.1.1	Production
4.1.2	Quality Control
4.1.3	Quality Assurance
4.1.4	Research & Development
4.1.5	Formulation Development
4.1.6	Purchase & Inventory Management
4.1.7	Regulatory Affairs
4.1.8	Executive- Training/ HR
4.1.9	Packaging

Hierarchy in Pharmaceutical Industry

The following hierarchy is usually found in Pharmaceutical industry. However it may vary from company to company.

⇨	**CHAIRMAN**
⇧	**PRESIDENT**
⇧	**SR. VICE PRESIDENT**
⇧	**VICE PRESIDENT**
⇧	**GENERAL MANAGER**
⇧	**DEPUTY GENERAL MANAGER**
⇧	**ASSIATANT GENERAL MANAGER**
⇧	**SR.MANAGER**
⇧	**MANAGER**
⇧	**DEPUTY MANAGER**
⇧	**ASST. MANAGER**
⇧	**SR. EXECUTIVE**
⇧	**EXECUTIVE**
⇧	**SR. OFFICER**
⇧	**OFFICER**
⇨	**TRAINEE OFFICER**

4.1.1 Production

This department produces pharmaceutical components and products like tablets, capsules, ointments, liquids etc. by setting-up, cleaning, operating and maintaining equipment, following aseptic procedures and documenting actions.

Job Description:

- Prepares for production by reviewing production schedule; studying and clarifying specifications; calculating requirements; assembling and weighing materials and supplies.
- Prepares equipment by performing sterile cleaning-in-place (CIP), servicing-in-place (SIP), and cleaning out-of-place (COP); conducting operator inspections; performing preventive maintenance checks.
- Produces requirements by operating and monitoring equipment; observing varying conditions; adjusting equipment controls; calculating concentrations, dilutions and yields; adhering to aseptic filtering and filing procedures.
- Maintains safe and clean work environment by following current good manufacturing practices (cGMP) and standard operating procedures; complying with legal regulations; monitoring environment.
- Keeps equipment operating by following operating instructions; troubleshooting breakdowns; calling for repairs.
- Documents production by completing forms, reports, logs and records of equipment and batches.
- Updates job knowledge by participating in training opportunities.
- Enhances organization reputation by accepting ownership for accomplishing new and different requests; exploring opportunities to add value to job accomplishments.

Profile Needed:

- Bachelor of Pharmacy with adequate knowledge on Equipment Calibration.
- Good Manufacturing Practice ().
- Manufacturing Methods and Procedures.
- Manufacturing Quality.
- Production Planning.
- Tooling.
- Pharmaceutics.
- Thoroughness.
- Documentation Skills.
- Analyzing Information.

Minimum of 2-4 years experience in Production department in the Pharmaceutical Manufacturing Industry is must for Supervisory/Senior Position

4.1.2 Quality Control (QC)

This department tests the quality of Raw Material, In-process intermediates and finished Active Pharmaceutical Ingredients (API) as per their specification.

Job Description:

- Testing of raw material, in-process, intermediate and finished active pharmaceutical ingredients (API) as per their specification.
- Calculating analytical data and entering the results in the note book for raw materials, in process, intermediates and finished active pharmaceutical ingredients (API) as per the written protocol.
- Preparation of Analytical Report as per the written protocol for in-process samples and for intermediates.
- Documentation, equipment maintenance, calibration, validation and handling customer complaints.
- Current good manufacturing practices (cGMP) compliance.
- Analytical method development, method validation, stability testing.
- Coordination with all departments regarding documentation requirements.

Profile Needed:

- The candidate should be a B. Pharm or M. Pharm (Pharmaceutical Analysis).
- Should have sound knowledge in handling QC equipments like UV, HPLC, GC, Karl Fisher etc. Analytical lab testing of raw materials, chemicals, intermediates and finished goods.
- Should have sound knowledge of principles of current good manufacturing practices (cGMP) and quality aspects.
- Minimum of 2-4 years experience in Quality Control department in the Pharmaceutical Intermediates/API/Bulk Drug Manufacturing Industry is must for higher posts.

4.1.3 Quality Assurance (QA)

This department assures the overall quality.

Job Description:

- To manage overall quality and compliance activities of product development life cycle.
- To ensure Product development activities are in compliance with regulations. To provide QA / Compliance support for product sustainment team for new product launches.
- To implement and maintain Industry's good manufacturing practice (GMP) quality manual from compliance perspective in order to establish appropriate corrective and preventive actions.
- To provide support during internal and external (HA) audits and to ensure all corrective actions are addressed as per designated timelines in development activities.

Profile Needed:

- Bachelor or Master of Pharmacy.
- Good communication, planning and organization skills.
- In depth understanding of pharmaceutical manufacturing, regulatory constraints.
- Validation and product development.
- Excellent analytical, organizational, and problem solving skills.
- Good knowledge of computer systems, i.e. Microsoft, Word, Excel & PowerPoint.
- Capable to manage multiple projects and deadlines.

4.1.4 Research & Development

Job Description:

- Leading R&D efforts of company from its inception to develop a range of new drugs and medical device products which may include Drug discovery, reverse engineering, formulation and process development, up scaling from pilot to manufacture, troubleshooting, stability, packaging development.
- Building and implementing a detailed laboratory research work plan to fulfill company's research objectives.
- Working to improve and expand company's formulation.
- Developing different range of products based on company's technology.
- Managing multi-disciplinary and multi-site teams to develop several products in parallel.
- Hosting audits from third parties and regulatory agencies.

Profile Needed:

- M Pharm or Ph D in Pharmacy.
- Proven scientific and technical ability to design and execute experimental studies as well as statistically analyze the data, author and review protocols and reports and present data.
- Excellent analytical, technical writing, communication and data management skills.
- An inquiring inquisitive mind, intense curiosity, and strong desire to innovate in the pharmaceuticals field.
- A strong grasp of current good manufacturing practices (cGMP) standards and requirements in FDA and EU regulated industries.
- Proven experience as a project manager with good supervisory and teamwork skills in a challenging environment (for higher posts).

4.1.5 Formulation Development

Job Description:

- Formulation design, development, optimization and scale up of oral, semi solid, solid and parenteral.
- Prepare laboratory prototype formulations and conduct systematic experiments to evaluate new types of formulation components.
- Write technical reports & procedures for experimental studies and laboratory related issue.
- Indian Pharmacopeia (IP) review of the molecule.
- Provide scientific guidance to technical staff when appropriate.

Profile Needed:

- M Pharm or Ph D in Pharmacy.
- Proven scientific and technical ability to design and execute experimental studies as well as statistically analyze the data, author and review protocols and reports and present data.
- Excellent analytical, technical writing, communication and data management skills.
- Knowledgeable with current good manufacturing practices (cGMP) and regulatory requirements for pharmaceuticals.
- Statistical data analysis knowledge

4.1.6 Purchase & Inventory Management

Job Description:

- To manage the activities of purchasing and inventory control departments and purchase supplies and materials at the optimal price and delivery cycle while maintaining lowest possible inventory levels.

Profile Needed:

- Bachelor of Pharmacy.
- Should have sound knowledge in purchase & inventory management.

4.1.7 Regulatory Affairs

Job Description:

- Ensuring that a company's products comply with the regulations of the Regulatory Agency like MHRA (Medicines and Healthcare Products Regulatory Agency), FDA (Food and Drug Administration) etc.
- Ensuring that guidelines and former practices of the importing country/buyer nation along with international legislations are adhered to.

- Collecting, collating and evaluating scientific data that has been researched by colleagues.
- Developing and writing clear arguments and explanations for new product licenses and license renewals.
- Preparing submissions of license variations and renewals to strict deadlines.
- Monitoring and setting timelines for license variations and renewal approvals.
- Working with specialist computer software and resources.
- Writing clear, accessible product labels and patient information leaflets.
- Planning and developing product trials and interpreting trial data.
- Advising scientists and manufacturers on regulatory requirements.
- Providing strategic advice to senior management throughout the development of a new product.
- Undertaking and managing regulatory inspections.
- Reviewing company practices and providing advice on changes to systems.
- Liaising with, and making presentations toregulatory authorities.
- Negotiating with regulatory authorities for marketing authorization.
- Specifying storage, labeling and packaging requirements.

Profile Needed:
- B.Pharm / M.Pharm preferably with knowledge on Regulatory requirements of different countries.

4.1.8 Executive- Training/ HR

Job Description:
- To undertake training need analysis for identification of training topics with respect to technical & soft skills/behavioral topics.
- To conduct induction & shop floor training sessions for new recruits.
- Follow up sessions on Standard Operating Procedure (SOP) Training as and when SOPs are changed.
- To conduct refresher training on ICH guidelines.
- To maintain training records for each employee on on-going basis.
- To develop tools to check the training effectiveness for the trainings imparted in recent past.
- To develop & regularly update a databank of technical questions & answers which would be used in test papers/discussion/brainstorming sessions to be evaluated by concerned SMEs (subject matter experts).

Profile Needed:

- B.Pharm / M.Pharm with additional qualification in MBA (operations management/ HR/ Training).

4.1.9 Packaging

Job Description:

- Packaging is a co-ordinated system of containment, transport, information and sale which ensures that the product reaches the user with claimed quality standards within the given shelf life.

Profile Needed:

- B.Pharm/ M.Pharm preferably with knowledge on Packaging.

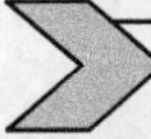
4.2 Pharmaceutical Marketing

Pharmaceutical marketing, sometimes called medico-marketing or pharma marketing is the business of advertising or otherwise promoting the sale of pharmaceuticals or drugs.

Few posts of Pharmaceutical Marketing are as follows

4.2.1	Marketing Manager
4.2.2	Product Manager
4.2.3	Product Executive
4.2.4	Medical Sales Representative
4.2.5	Area Manager
4.2.6	Regional Manager
4.2.7	Zonal Manager

4.2.1 Marketing Manager

Job Description:

- To lead market growth and penetration through implementation of comprehensive marketing plans and training and sales support materials supporting the distribution partners to drive sales.

- To help execute a Strategic Sales Business Plan which includes lead generation, sales planning, marketing strategies, delivery of pre- and post-sales support, training and development of distributors.

- To manage the mix of product sales and ensure that the full portfolio of products and services is marketed and sold effectively.

- To ensure competitive strategies are current and understood by sales, marketing, service and clinical teams.

Profile Needed:

- B. Pharm
- Marketing creativity and ability to take risks and ask the right questions.
- Self-driven and motivated and have uncompromising honesty and ethics.

4.2.2 Product Manager

Job Description:

- To provide the sales team with the necessary technical expertise to enable them to sell the product. This involves printed and electronic promotional material, product training, and relevant clinical papers.
- To review product data to ensure that the field force is kept up to date on new developments regarding the companies or competitors products.
- To act as point of first reference for all products related enquiries and work collaboratively with colleagues in Clinical Research and Regulatory to address any issues that may arise.
- To assess the response and suitability of current promotional material and to ensure that the printed promotional material is being used optimally.
- To design market research projects to assess customer attitudes to the current product range and new product introductions.
- To assist with the development of the annual marketing plan and for controlling advertising, promotion and sales aids in accordance with the annual marketing plan.
- To prepare product forecasts, and constantly monitoring inventory levels held at central and interstate warehouses including liaison with production (locally and globally) to ensure supply timelines.
- Liaise with the advertising agency regarding the product campaign including journal advertising, direct mail and conferences.

Profile Needed:

- Bachelor of Pharmacy.
- Managing budgets (for catering, outside speakers, conferences, hospitality, etc.)
- Good communication, planning, and organization skills.

4.2.3 Product Executive

Job Description:

- Planning and developing the marketing strategy for fast moving over the counter products.
- Yearly budgeting and quarterly sales and marketing management.
- New product identification and new launch.
- Carrying out brand building activities.
- Training and supporting field personnel, enchasing customer relationships.
- Brief and train the sales force.
- Analyzing Market Trends & Creating Winning Strategies.

Profile Needed:

- Bachelor of Pharmacy.
- Good communication, planning and organization skills.
- Must have handled products in acute therapy.

4.2.4 Medical Sales Representative

Medical sales representatives (widely referred to as reps) are a key link between medical and pharmaceutical companies and healthcare professionals. They sell their company's products which include medicines, prescription drugs and medical equipment to a variety of customers including General Practitioners (GP), Primary Care Trusts (PCTs), Hospitals and Pharmacies. They also work strategically to increase the awareness and use of their company's Pharmaceutical and medical products.

Post: Medical Representative

Hierarchy:

The following hierarchy is usually found in Pharmaceutical marketing. However it may vary from company to company.

⇨	**Managing Director**
⇧	**Chairman**
⇧	**Vice President**
⇧	**International Sales Manager**
⇧	**National Sales Manager**
⇧	**Zonal Sales Manager**
⇧	**Regional Manager**
⇧	**Area Manager**
⇨	**Medical Representative**

Job Description:

- To arrange appointments with doctors, pharmacists and hospital medical teams which may include pre-arranged appointments or regular 'cold' calling.
- Making presentations to doctors, practice staff and nurses in GP surgeries, hospital doctors and pharmacists in the retail sector. Presentations may take place in medical settings during the day, or may be conducted in the evenings at a local hotel or conference venue.
- To organize conferences for doctors and other medical staff.
- Building and maintaining positive working relationships with medical staff and supporting administrative staff.

- To manage budgets (for catering, outside speakers, conferences, hospitality, etc.).
- To keep detail records of all contacts.
- Reaching (and if possible exceeding) annual sales targets.
- To plan work schedules and weekly and monthly timetables. This may involve working with the area sales team or discussing future targets with the area sales manager. Generally, medical sales executives have their own regional area of responsibility and plan how and when to target health professionals.
- Regularly attending company meetings, technical data presentations and briefings.
- To keep up-to-date latest clinical data supplied by the company, and interpreting, presenting and discussing this data with health professionals during presentations.
- To monitor competitor activity and competitors' products.
- To develop strategies for increasing opportunities to meet and talk to contacts in the medical and healthcare sector.

Profile Needed:
- Bachelor of Pharmacy.
- Good communication, planning, and organization skills.
- In depth understanding of marketing.
- Excellent analytical, organizational, and problem solving skills.
- Good knowledge of computer systems, i.e. Microsoft, Word, Excel & PowerPoint.

4.2.5 Area Manager

Job Description:
- To monitor and analyzing market trends.
- To study competitors' products and services.
- To explore ways of improving existing products and services, and increasing profitability.
- To identify target markets and developing strategies to communicate with them.
- To prepare and manage marketing plans and budgets.
- To manage the production of promotional material.
- To liaison with other internal departments such as sales and distribution.
- Producing reports to monitor results.

- Presenting findings and suggestions to company directors or other senior managers.
- Travelling to trade shows, conferences and sales meetings.
- To support and manage a marketing team.

Profile Needed:

- Bachelor of Pharmacy or other Scientific Disciplines.
- Good communication, planning, and organization skills.
- Having 3 to 4 years experience as a Medical Representative.
- Excellent analytical, organizational, and problem solving skills.
- Good knowledge of computer systems, i.e. Microsoft, Word, Excel & PowerPoint.

4.2.6 Regional Manager

Job Description:

- Provides quality leadership for company's internal and external customers in all assigned tasks, while upholdincompany values at all times: inclusive of constructive problem solving, facilitating creative improvements, and inspiring others. Achieves the region's revenue and profitability quotas for company products as they are sold into all customer segments within region. Establishes an environment and foundation for future sales growth. Sells and teaches others how to sell value and solutions to company's customers.
- Directs the selling activities within the region, inclusive of resource deployment and customer interactions. Prioritizes effectively and in accordance with corporate objectives.
- Efficiently manages the region's Hospital, Professional Education, Government and distribution relationships.
- Leads the sales territory representatives and specialists, inclusive of managing performance, coaching, mentoring, hiring and career development.
- Responsible for the region's forecasting and sales tracking.
- Sets the vision for the region and develops and adheres to a business plan to attain this vision.
- Evaluate market trends and gather competitive information, identify trends that effect current and future growth of regional sales and profitability. Disseminate information to regional sales representatives, corporate marketing and sales operations.
- Special projects as assigned.

- Empowered to make decisions within the region and on behalf of the region, and authority to make cross functional decisions in partnership with peers of other functions.

Profile Needed:

- Bachelor's degree in Pharmacy, life sciences or business (preferred) and three years sales management experience.
- Proven leadership skills.
- Supervisory or management experience, preferably of a sales staff.
- Working knowledge of healthcare, medical education market segments within an assigned sales territory.
- Demonstrated record of achievement in a prior sales position.
- Strong closing skills.
- Proven oral, written, telephone and presentation skills. Strong interpersonal skills.
- Ability to learn and retain product specific information and utilize to position the features and benefits to customers.
- Computer literate with knowledge of all Microsoft Office Applications especially Excel.

4.2.7 Zonal Manager

Job Description:

- Manpower Recruitment to fill up all existing vacancies or vacancies arising out of expansion plan within a reasonable period of time.
- Training & Development of the team member both classroom and in field (On Job Training) to achieve better result and to prepare them to take higher responsibilities in future as when the need arises.
- To develop the team spirit among Regional Sales Manager (RSM), Area Sales Manager (ASM) and Medical Representatives.
- To guide and assist RSM, ASM and Medical Representative in their respective territories and to enable them to achieve targets both product wise, unit wise as well as rupee value wise.
- To ensure implementation of marketing strategies for the promotion of the product and also field related strategies in the zone.
- To monitor the work done by the team members and advice measures to bring out an improvement in the quality of the field work in order to produce higher result.
- To ensure maintenance of healthy relationship with the distributors, core doctors, with the team and carry out activities to nurture and grow in the interest of the organization.

- To coordinate with logistic/distribution department in consultation with the managers from time to time to ensure that stocks are made available at C&F and at distributors point.
- To ensure the clearance of outstanding/overdue of the distributors with regular follow up through team members.
- Settlement of claims of distributors by coordinating with logistics/distribution department in consultation with the managers from time to time.
- To ensure coverage of institutional customers and all team members and maintains a personal touch with them for continuity of existing business and procurement of new business.
- To continuously guide the team members to resolve their problems in course of their day to day field work.
- To ensure effective communication with regard to the policies, procedures etc. of the company to the team members.
- To handle the regular correspondence of the team members by acknowledging their letters and answering their queries.
- To participate in the Conferences/Cycle meets/ Marketing meetings/review meeting held with the Sales, Marketing/Product team and give suggestions for effective marketing strategy.
- Periodical appraisal of team members.
- To provide feedback to the Senior Management on all the activities of self, team and seek advice for continuous improvement.

Profile Needed:
- Bachelor's degree in Pharmacy, life sciences or business (preferred).
- Proven leadership skills.
- Supervisory or management experience, preferably of a sales staff.
- Working knowledge of healthcare, medical education market segments within an assigned sales territory.
- Demonstrated record of achievement in a prior sales position.
- Strong closing skills. Proven oral, written, telephone and presentation skills. Strong interpersonal skills.
- Ability to learn and retain product specific information and utilize to position the features and benefits to customers.
- Knowledge of human anatomy and physiology.
- Computer literate with knowledge of all Microsoft Office Applications especially Excel.

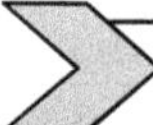 **4.3 Drug Administration (State & Central)**

To regulate the Drug Administration department of State & Central Government

Few posts under this category are as follows

4.3.1	Drugs Inspector
4.3.2	Drugs Controller
4.3.3	Official in Central Drug Control Laboratory
4.3.4	Official in State Drug Control Laboratory
4.3.5	Scientific Officer
4.3.6	Government Analyst

4.3.1 Drugs Inspector

Drugs Inspector is a lucrative career option for aspirants who have completed their Bachelors degree in Pharmacy. They can get into the post of Drugs Inspector based on their performance in written test, viva voce and physical fitness. They may need few years experience in the manufacturing field as well. The recruitment to the position of Drugs Inspector is conducted by UPSC and also various state PSCs on an annual basis.

Post: Drugs Inspector

Hierarchy:

	Drugs Controller (of the concerned State)
	Deputy Drugs Controller (DDC)
	Assistant Drugs Controller (ADC)
	Drugs Inspector (DI)

Job Description:

- Inspects establishment where foods, drugs, cosmetics and similar consumer items are manufactured, handled, stored or sold and to enforce legal standards of sanitation, purity and grading.
- Visit specified establishments to investigate sanitary conditions and health and hygiene habits of persons handling consumer products.
- Collect samples of products for bacteriological and chemical laboratory analysis.
- Destroys samples or prohibits sale of impure, toxic, damaged or misbranded items.
- Inform individuals concerned of specific regulations affecting establishments.
- Questions employees, vendors, consumers etc to obtain evidence for prosecuting violators of drug regulations.

- Ascertains that required licenses and permits have been obtained and are displayed.
- Prepares reports on each establishment visited, including findings and recommendations for action Negotiate with marketers and processors to effect changes in facilities and practices, where undesirable conditions are discovered that are not specifically prohibited by law.
- Grade products according to specified standards.
- Test products, using variety of specialized test equipments, such as ultraviolet lights and filter.
- Investigate compliance with or violation of public sanitation laws and regulations and be designated Sanitary Inspector.

Profile Needed:

- Aspirants should hold a Bachelor's degree in Pharmacy.

4.3.2 Drugs Controller

Job Description:

- To render technical advice to Government and other Heads of Departments on matters relating to the enforcement of Drugs and Cosmetics Act 1940 and Drugs and Cosmetics Rules 1945.
- Budget of State Drugs Control Administration.
- Enforcing Drugs and Magic Remedies Act.
- Enforcing Dangerous Drugs Act and the state Manufacturing Drug Rules.
- Enforcing the Drug Price Control Over 1979.
- To render technical advice to Government and other Heads of Departments on matters relating to the enforcement of Dangerous Drugs Act, Medicinal and Toilet preparation (Excise duties) Act, prohibition Act, Poison Act.
- Guidance to the Drug Inspectors in ensuring that the Provisions of different drug acts are enforced.

Profile Needed:

- The candidate should be a Pharmacy graduate preferably with knowledge on different Drug Acts.
- Experience (as per Govt. norms) as a Drugs Inspector/ ADC/ DDC.

4.3.3 Official in Central Drug Control Laboratory

Central Drug Testing Laboratory (CDTL) Mumbai, is the regulatory laboratory of the Ministry of Health & Family Welfare, Government of India working under the administrative control of the Drugs Controller General (India), Central Drugs Standardization Control Organization (CDSCO), and DGHS.

Job Description:

- Testing of import and export bulk drugs, formulations & Cosmetics referred by Port Authorities of Mumbai, Ahmdabad, New Delhi, Kolkata & Chennai.
- Testing of survey and watcher samples sent by Deputy Drug Controllers (All 4 zones).
- Quality Testing of New Drug samples submitted to Drugs Controller General (India) for approval for manufacture and sale in the country.
- Samples submitted for site registration as intimated by Drugs Controller General (India).
- Testing of field samples of Oral Contraceptive Pills, Copper T & tubal rings sent by Department of Family Welfare, Ministry of Health & Family Welfare.

Profile Needed:

- The candidate should be a Pharmacy graduate with in depth knowledge on different Drug Acts.

4.3.4 Official in State Drug Control Laboratory

Job Description:

- **Coding:** Coding of received samples and distribution to other analytical division for analysis.
- **Chemical I:** Analysis of Bulk Drug & Drug Formulations like liquid oral products, ointments, creams, lotions, gels etc.
- **Chemical II:** Analysis of Drug Formulations like tablets and capsules except Antibiotics and Vitamins.
- **Antibiotics:** Analysis of Antibiotic Formulations.
- **Vitamins:** Analysis of Vitamins and nutritional supplement formulations.
- **Pharmacology:** Analysis of Ophthalmic, Large volume/Small Volume parenteral preparations, Intramuscular / Intravenous injectables.
- **Pharmacognosy:** Analysis of Ayurvedic Drugs and Surgical dressings.
- **Cosmetics:** Analysis of cosmetic products.

Profile Needed:

- The candidate should be a Pharmacy graduate preferably with knowledge on different Drug Acts.

4.3.5 Scientific Officer

Job Description:

- Primary job duties include devising research proposals and programs based on the desires of the organization's executives.

- Scientific officers also supervise the implementation of those programs and coordinate the work between different labs and phases of the research for maximum efficiency and progress.

- Scientific officers then report these results to executives. They may also meet with clients or regulators to discuss report or explain projects.

- Integral secondary job duties include hiring personnel, training them for the specific research projects and supervising their research.

- Scientific officers must also manage the budget for their division, including personnel salaries, equipment and supply costs.

- Additionally, they develop acceptable work policies and procedures that meet government or industry regulatory standards.

Profile Needed:

- The candidate should be a Pharmacy graduate / B. Sc Biological or Life Science degree and Higher Welfare Science Degree (veterinary).

4.3.6 Government Analyst

A government analyst job can be very challenging and rewarding, particularly for those who enjoy being intellectually engaged and have high analytical Skills. Analysts should also be very strong in the areas of analysis, evaluation methods and program assessing techniques.

Job Description:

- An analyst gathers, records, and analyzes data that pertains to a specific agency, program, or project.

- He or she may track policy development or watch legislative movement within a particular field.

- He or she should also know the agency policies, mission and objectives as well as management processes and principles.

- Depending upon the area of analysis, some are required to possess and comprehend financial management practices or basic budgetary principles.

Profile Needed:

- The candidate should be a Pharmacy graduate from any recognized institution of State or Central Government with experience as Scientific Officer as per government norms.

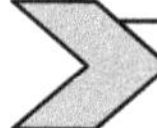

4.4 Entrepreneurship

The capacity and willingness to develop, organize and manage a business venture along with its risks in order to make a profit. The most obvious example of entrepreneurship is the starting of new businesses. In economics, entrepreneurship combined with land, labor, natural resources and capital can produce profit. Entrepreneurial spirit is characterized by innovation and risk-taking, and is an essential part of a nation's ability to succeed in an ever changing and increasingly competitive global marketplace.

- A Bachelor of Pharmacy can establish his/her own Pharmaceutical Industry.
- Own a Retail or Wholesale Medicine Shop.

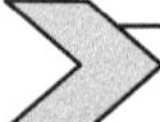

4.5 Academics

After completion of B Pharm or M Pharm you can start your career in academics also.

After B. Pharm
- Teacher in D. Pharm Institutes
- Higher studies (M Pharm & Pharm D)
- Higher Studies Abroad (MS)
- Post Graduate in Business Management

After M. Pharm
- Teacher in B. Pharm Institutes
- May Pursue Ph. D

After Pharm. D
- Teacher in B. Pharm/M. Pharm Institutes
- May Pursue Ph.D

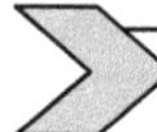

4.6 Clinical Research

Clinical research is a branch of medical science that determines the safety and effectiveness of medications, devices, diagnostic products and treatment regimens intended for human use. These may be used for prevention, treatment, diagnosis or for relieving symptoms of a disease. Clinical Research is different from clinical practice. In clinical practice, one use established treatments while in clinical research evidence is collected to establish a treatment.

Few posts under this category are as follows

4.6.1   Clinical Research Associate (CRA)

4.6.2	Clinical Research Coordinator (CRC)
4.6.3	Clinical Data Coordinator (CDC)
4.6.4	Clinical Logistics Leader (CLL)
4.6.5	Biostatician

4.6.1 Clinical Research Associate (CRA)

Job Description:

- Developing and writing trial protocols (outlining the purpose and methodology of a trial).
- Presenting trial protocols to a steering committee.
- Designing data collection forms, known as case report forms (CRFs).
- Coordinating with the ethics committee which safeguards the rights, safety and wellbeing of all trial subjects.
- Managing regulatory authority applications and approvals that oversee the research and marketing of new and existing drugs.
- Identifying and assessing the suitability of facilities to be used as the clinical trial site.
- Identifying/selecting an investigator who will be responsible for the conduct of the trial at the trial site.
- Liaising with doctors/consultants or investigators on conducting the trial.
- Setting up the trial sites which include ensuring each centre has the trial materials, including the trial drug often known as the investigational medicinal product. Training the site staff to trial-specific industry standards.
- Monitoring the trial throughout its duration which involves visiting the trial sites on a regular basis.
- Verifying that data entered on to the CRFs is consistent with patient clinical notes known as source data/document verification (SDV).
- Collecting completed CRFs from hospitals and general practices.
- Writing visit reports.
- Filing and collating trial documentation and reports.
- Ensuring accountability and maintaining records for all unused trial supplies
- Closing down trial sites on completion of the trial.
- Discussing results with a medical statistician, who usually writes technical trial reports.
- Archiving study documentation and correspondence.
- Preparing final reports and occasionally manuscripts for publication.

Profile Needed:

- Bachelor's Degree in Pharmacy, Healthcare or Clinical Research related field preferred.
- Certified Clinical Research Coordinator (CCRC) or Certified Clinical Research Associate (CCRA) preferred.
- Proficient in word processing, computer spreadsheets, mainframe computer applications, and database management.

4.6.2 Clinical Research Coordinator (CRC)

Plan, direct, or coordinate clinical research projects. Direct the activities of workers engaged in clinical research projects to ensure compliance with protocols and overall clinical objectives. May evaluate and analyze clinical data.

Job Description:

- Serves as primary study coordinator for research protocols at affiliated hospitals or in the outpatient clinic setting as assigned by Director.
- Directs the conduct of clinical studies to ensure adherence to the research protocol and provides bimonthly updates to Principal Investigator on study progress.
- Screens patient records, databases, and physician referral summaries for identification of prospective candidates for research protocols.
- Interview prospective subjects for participation in investigations and obtains informed consent.
- Participates in initiation visits/investigator's meetings for assigned clinical trials (may involve travel) and implements these trials according to a deadline schedule mutually agreed upon by PI and sponsor.
- Develops study working folders for assigned protocols to outline guidelines for protocol compliance and to assure complete source documentation.
- Educates human subjects for participation in investigations.
- Educates clinic/hospital personnel for participation in protocol conduct, data collection process, and related conceptual issues as applicable.
- Maintains consistent enrollment in protocols and provides monthly written documentation of screening/enrollment/follow-up activities.
- Coordinates the collection of data according to the research protocol, operations manual, and case report form guidelines within the budgetary guidelines established by Director.
- Draws, prepares, and ships laboratory samples for clinical trials.
- Maintains investigational drug/device dispensing accountability and shipping logs according to protocol guidelines.

- Performs electrocardiogram (ECG/EKG, Holter monitoring, physical exams, and other procedures as directed by study protocol.

- Discuss with Principal Investigator on procedures and tests that need to be performed in compliance with the study protocol and updates Principal Investigator on the results of procedures and tests.

- Documents research related examinations, procedures, tests, and other activities in appropriate clinic or hospital charts.

- Completes phone logs for conversations with sponsors, patients, physicians and coordinating organizations.

- Schedules follow-up visits for study patients in collaboration with Principal Investigator and provides source documentation for the activities conducted during these visits.

- Completes accurate and complete data entry into case report forms or pre-established computer programmed formats ensuring appropriate source documentation.

- Schedules and undergoes sponsor initiated monitor visits and quality assurance audits for periodic reviewing and querying of collected data in a timely fashion.

- Identifies strategies to improve patient enrollment in research protocols in collaboration with Principal Investigator.

Profile Needed:

- Bachelor's or Master's Degree in Pharmacy, Healthcare or Clinical Research related field preferred.

- Certified Clinical Research Coordinator (CCRC) or Certified Clinical Research Associate (CCRA), preferred.

- Proficient in word processing, computer spreadsheets, mainframe computer applications, and database management.

- Ability to prioritize and organize a high volume workload and changing priorities.

- Familiar with principles of protocol development, study design, statistics, and IRB process.

4.6.3 Clinical Data Coordinator (CDC)

Job Description:

- The Sr. Clinical Data Coordinator provides comprehensive data management expertise to Data Management.

- The position also requires providing efficient, quality data management products that meet customer needs. Provide leadership either in the role of the Data Operations Coordinator (DOC), or in a leadership role in a specific Department task.

- Serve as Data Operations Coordinator (DOC) for one or two global studies with fewer than 10 operations staff, or serve in a leadership role to a specific data management Task.
- Manage delivery of projects through full data management study life-cycle (with minimal guidance).
- Manage project timelines (with guidance from DTL or Manager).
- Management of quality (with guidance from DTL or Manager).
- Determining resource needs (with guidance from DTL or Manager).
- Identify Out of Scope Work.
- Serve as back-up for Data Operations Coordinator or Data Team Lead (with guidance).
- Perform comprehensive data management tasks including data review, writing and resolving data clarifications.
- Perform database designer activities for technologies not requiring extensive programming.
- Perform comprehensive quality control procedures.
- Independently bring project solutions to the CDM team.
- Solves issues through using global issue escalation/communication plan.
- Consult with Standards Group for process issues; communicate ideas for process improvement.
- Assist in developing and implementing new technology.
- Understand and comply with core operating procedures and working instructions.
- Perform other duties as directed by the Data Operations Coordinator, Group Manager.
- Meet objectives as assigned.
- Develop and maintain good communications and working relationships with CDM team.
- Interact with CDM team members to negotiate timelines and responsibilities.

Profile Needed:

- A Bachelor's/ Master's degree (preferably in Pharmacy, Health Sciences, Science or Clinical).
- Other relevant degree with minimum 1-2 years of relevant work experience (clinical trials experience in function similar to DM) and a total work experience of at least 4 years.
- A background in Medical Terminology, Pharmacology, Anatomy, and Physiology required for many tasks.

- The position expects excellent organizational, communication, and data management skills.
- Able to make independent decisions within scope of authority and considers the impact of decisions on other groups/people.
- Basic understanding of Drug Development Process and its relevance to Data Management.

4.6.4 Clinical Logistics Leader (CLL)

Job Description:

- Lead the Clinical Logistics Services teams by combining a depth of clinical logistics experience with insight into client pressures and an ability to develop the right solution for the client.
- This requires a vast business understanding in order to make effective decisions independently and the knowledge and experience required to confidently recommending a course of action.
- This includes providing the overall CLS functional leadership of clinical trials or clinical programs and the Clinical Logistics Services teams to achieve operational excellence; and
- Delivering projects / programs on time, to budget, to the highest quality, compliant with ICH GCP, exceeding client expectations.
- This position is responsible for the profitability of managed CLS project(s) and client satisfaction.

Profile Needed:

- Master degree, or equivalent (e.g. Pharm. D.), in biology, pharmacy, or
- Other health-related discipline, international trade, business administration or
- Logistics with pharmaceutical/clinical research/consulting industry experience.

4.6.5 Biostatician

Job Description:

- Assist with or lead biostatistics projects with low to moderate complexity.
- Assist in the process of protocol development by choosing appropriate study designs, including statistical methodologies.
- Write and review Statistical Analysis Plans (SAPs) based on protocol including development of well-presented mock-up displays for tables, listings, and figures.
- Participate in project teams as biostatistics representative, and support business development meetings by attending sponsor bid defense meetings.

- Conduct verification and quality control of project deliverables, ensuring that output meets expected results and is consistent with analysis described in SAP.
- Create or review programming specifications for analysis of datasets, tables, listings, and figures.
- Generate randomization schedule ensuring no errors are present and sponsor and protocol requirements are met.

Profile Needed:

- Bachelor's or Master's or Ph.D degree in Pharmacy.
- Biostatistics, Public health or related experience.
- Demonstrated knowledge or experience with clinical trials.
- SAS programming.
- Statistical design and analysis methodology.
- Statistical theory including experimental design.
- Categorical data analysis.
- Analysis of variance (covariance).
- Survival analysis, and non-parametric methods.
- Application of basic statistical design, analysis.
- ICH guidelines.
- Programming techniques utilized in clinical research, and
- Communication of statistical concepts required.

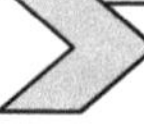 ## 4.7 Hospital (Govt. & Private)

Pharmacy is an essential part of Health Care system. There are several posts in the Health Care System. Those are as follows

4.7.1	Hospital Pharmacist
4.7.2	Clinical Pharmacist
4.7.3	Prescription Audit Team (PAT)
4.7.4	Pharmacy Store In-charge
4.7.5	Procurement Officer
4.7.6	Purchase & Inventory Management
4.7.7	Pharmacovigilance officer in CDSCO (Govt.)
4.7.8	Pharmacist cum Logistic Asst. (NRHM)
4.7.9	Emergency Medical Technician (Ambulance)
4.7.10	Multipurpose Health Worker
4.7.11	Health Advice Officer

4.7.1 Hospital Pharmacist

Job Description: Checking prescriptions to ensure that there are no errors and that they are appropriate and safe for the individual patient;

- Providing advice on the dosage of medicines and the most appropriate form of medication, for example, tablet, injection, ointment or inhaler.
- Participating in ward rounds, taking patient drug histories and involvement in decision-making on appropriate treatments.
- Discussing treatments with patients' relatives, Community Pharmacists and Physians.
- Ensuring medicines are stored appropriately and securely.
- Supervising the work of less experienced and less qualified staff.
- Answering questions about medicines from within the hospital, other hospitals and the general public.
- Keeping up to date with, and contributing to, research and development.
- Writing guidelines for drug use within the hospital and implementing hospital regulations.
- Providing information on expenditure on drugs.
- Preparing and quality-checking sterile medications, for example, intravenous medications.
- Setting up and supervising clinical trials.

Profile Needed:

- Bachelor's Degree in Pharmacy/Diploma in Pharmacy/ Bachelor's degree in Pharmacy Practice.
- Certifications in different areas of Pharmacy and an accredited residence program are a plus.
- However, certain personal abilities are all vital, such as communication abilities (both oral and written), deep knowledge on drugs, medical procedures and therapies, diagnosis and disease states, and some pharmaco-kinetics.
- Skills in working with technical automated equipment and information systems are an added value to any Pharmacy Career.

4.7.2 Clinical Pharmacist

Job Description:

- Works with the pharmacy staff and management to acquire an understanding of the underlying needs of the department and translates these needs into how the system should be built.
- Develops and documents internal procedures.

- Prepares details of specifications as needed and understands choices in application specifications.
- Investigates preferred choices of users.
- Analyzes data conversion needs.
- A Clinical Pharmacist is in charge of providing various services to the Division Director, such as taking part in continuing education programs for Medical staff, health care services, and Pharmacy students, advising physicians on drug usage and dose control in hospitals and clinics, and assisting the Division Director in his everyday duties.

Profile Needed:

- B Pharm. Degree or a Doctor Pharmacy Degree and at least a two-years experience.
- Certifications in different areas of Pharmacy and an accredited residence program is a plus point.
- Skills in working with technical automated equipment and information systems are an added value to any Pharmacy Career.

4.7.3 Prescription Audit Team (PAT)

Prescription audit is an important mechanism to improve the quality of care afforded by the hospitals. Data generated on the morbidity pattern coupled with the current practices of treatment of these diseases provided an objective basis for preparing an Essential Medicines List (EML). Comparing the current usage of drugs with the standard treatment guidelines will enhance the effectiveness of treatment and render it cost-effective.

Job Description:

- Analyze the prescription.
- Thoroughly check the drug utilization pattern.
- Appropriate guidelines (about medicines) have to be given to the patients.

Profile Needed:

- Bachelor of Pharmacy/ Master of Pharmacy/ Pharm. D.

4.7.4 Pharmacy Store In-Charge

Job Description:

- Dispense and counsel medications.
- Assay radiopharmaceuticals, verify rates of disintegration, and calculate the volume required to produce the desired results, to ensure proper dosages.

- Manage pharmacy operations, hiring and supervising staff, performing administrative duties, and buying and selling non-pharmaceutical merchandise.
- Assess the identity, strength and purity of medications.

Profile Needed:

- Diploma in Pharmacy/ Bachelor of Pharmacy.
- Must be licensed to practice.

4.7.5 Procurement Officer

A procurement officer, also known as a purchasing manager, is an important person in any organization. He ensures that the company makes wise purchase of goods or services to resell or use. The demand for the services of purchasing managers has increased.

Job Description:

- Requests for Quotations (RFQ), use bid evaluation criteria and other competitive procurement tools to ensure client needs are met, and to ensure procurement processes are perceived by suppliers as fair, open and ethical.
- Analyses procurement requirements and selects the most appropriate methods based on interpretation and assessment of established policies, practices, and experience.
- Plans, organizes and leads the bid solicitation process including drafting and issuing RFQ, RFP, developing bid evaluation criteria and guiding clients on processes involved.
- Chairs bid evaluation committees, ensures the integrity of the competitive process, facilitates bidder debriefings, and exercises appropriate judgment and tact while ensuring to protect confidential information.
- Analyses, negotiates and prepares contractual agreements, ensuring appropriate terms and conditions.
- Monitors and reviews progress of contractual agreements, reviews and approves invoices for payment, resolves any problems that arise, performs post contract evaluations, creates and maintains procurement records, including electronic records in Enterprise Resource Planning (ERP) system, Oracle, and other systems, ensuring accuracy and integrity of data.
- Provides advice and guidance to clients on shipping methods and services, risks, and costs for domestic and international shipments, analyses logistical requirements and decides on appropriate methods and services to use, based on standard practice, and plans, executes and monitors shipments.

- Provides required written authorizations, and prepares/issues instructions and import/export documentation to suppliers, freight forwarders, and/or carriers, to ensure timely and safe arrival of goods, and compliance with domestic and international shipping regulations, Customs regulations etc., and takes necessary action to resolve problems/disputes.

Profile Needed:

- Bachelor's Degree in Pharmacy, Healthcare or related field preferred.
- Contract administration and / or procurement experience.

4.7.6 Purchase & Inventory Management

Job Description:

- Implement improvement processes and systems to reduce inventory, minimize costs and maximize working capital.
- Write and maintain accurate written procedures for all main inventory control processes and functions.
- Be responsible for managing and running planned stock takes.
- Perform cyclic stock checks.
- Check and adjust shop floor data collection data.
- Ensure works orders are correct and fully completed and that all stock has been allocated to the job correctly.
- Ensure integrity and accuracy of the stock management system.
- Produce daily reports to ensure key critical areas of the stock system are controlled and any discrepancies addressed and resolved.
- Manage control measures to ensure mistakes, inaccuracies and discrepancies are highlighted, addressed and resolved.

Profile Needed:

- Ideally possessing a relevant professional qualification (Pharmacy) and/or suitable background experience in inventory management / purchasing.
- Have a detailed understanding of MRP and inventory control / management systems and ERP.
- Strong analytical and problem solving skills.
- Experience of lean manufacture, kanban and kaizen continuous improvement or similar production tools within a low volume, high quality manufacturing facility would be an advantage.
- Possess excellent verbal and written communication skills for a demanding and customer focused working environment.
- Possess the willingness to learn, improve and adapt.

4.7.7 Pharmacovigilance Officer in CDSCO (Govt.)

Job Description:

- Preparation of the blueprint for collection, collation, analysis of ADR reports, received from various centers all over the country and implementation of the pharmacovigilance programme.
- Preparation of guidelines / documentation etc. for the programme.
- Co-ordination of spurious drugs survey at National Level. Any other duties assigned by Drugs Controller General of India (DCGI) from time to time.

Profile Needed:

Master degree in Pharmacy with Pharmacology or Clinical Pharmacy with some years experience in collation/ analysis of ADR reports.

4.7.8 Pharmacist Cum Logistic Asst. (NRHM)

The National Rural Health Mission (NRHM) was launched in April 2005. The NRHM focused especially on 18 states, with poor infrastructure and low public health indicators, namely the eight Empowered Action Group (EAG) states - (Bihar, Jharkhand, Madhya Pradesh, Chhattisgarh, Uttar Pradesh, Uttaranchal, Odisha and Rajasthan), the eight North Eastern States (Assam, Arunachal Pradesh, Manipur, Mizoram, Meghalaya, Nagaland, Sikkim, Tripura) and two other states, namely, Himachal Pradesh and Jammu & Kashmir.

Job Description:

- He/ she should take care of the logistics in additions to their job as a Pharmacist.

Profile Needed:

- Degree /Diploma in Pharmacy, minimum 1 year experience in managing a drug ware house in reputed hospital / health centre recognized by the Govt.

4.7.9 Emergency Medical Technician (Ambulance)

Job Description:

- Opening and maintaining an airway.
- Ventilating patients.
- Administering cardiopulmonary resuscitation, including use of automated external defibrillators.
- Providing pre hospital emergency medical care of simple and multiple system trauma such as:

  Controlling hemorrhage,

  - Treatment of shock (hypo perfusion),
  - Bandaging wounds,

- Immobilization of painful, swollen, or deformed extremities,
- Immobilization of painful, swollen, or deformed neck or spine.
- Providing emergency medical care to:
  - Assist in emergency childbirth,
  - Manage general medical complaints of altered mental status, respiratory, cardiac, diabetic, allergic reaction, seizures, poisoning behavioral emergencies, environmental emergencies, and psychological crises. Additional care is provided based upon assessment of the patient and obtaining historical information.
- Searching for medical identification emblems as a guide to appropriate emergency medical care.
- Assisting patients with prescribed medications, including sublingual nitroglycerin, epinephrine auto injectors and hand-held aerosol inhalers.
- Administration of oxygen, oral glucose and activated charcoal.
- Reassuring patients and bystanders by working in a confident, efficient manner.
- Avoiding mishandling and undue haste while working expeditiously to accomplish the task.

Profile Needed:
- Bachelor of Pharmacy/ Diploma in Pharmacy.

4.7.10 Multipurpose Health Worker

Job Description:
- MPHW (Male) should make a visit to each family once a month.
- He will mainly focus on activities which are related to disease control programs, detection and control of epidemic outbreaks, environmental sanitation, safe drinking water, first aid in emergencies like accidents, injuries, burns etc.
- Treatment of common/ minor illnesses, communication and counseling, life style diseases and logistics and supply management at sub-centre.
- In addition he will also help ANM in MCH, Family Welfare, and Nutrition related activities.

Profile Needed:
- D. Pharm / B. Pharm.

4.7.11 Health Advice Officer

Job Description:
- To provide Health Advice to patients with the help of doctors. For example: to advice diabetic patients about food & drug administration.

- To create awareness among the patients about use of medicines.
- Ready to work in rotational shifts.

Profile Needed:

- D. Pharm / B. Pharm / M. Pharm.

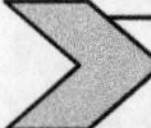 ## 4.8 IT & Insurance

After completion of B.Pharm or M.Pharm you may create your career in Information Technology (IT) & Insurance field also.

4.8.1	Medical Coding
4.8.2	Medical Transcription
4.8.3	Clinical Data Management
4.8.4	Pharmacovigilance
4.8.5	Prescription Data Base Maintenance
4.8.6	Patient Care Advisor
4.8.7	Quality Analyst
4.8.8	Software Development
4.8.9	Medical Claims Processors
4.8.10	SAS Programmer

4.8.1 Medical Coding

Job Description:

- Understand the client requirements and specifications of the project and Code the charts accordingly.
- Meet the productivity targets of clients within the stipulated time.
- Ensure that the deliverables to the client adhere to the quality standards.
- Prepare and maintain status reports.
- Statistical analysis of diseases and therapeutic actions.
- Reimbursement.
- Knowledge-based and decision support systems.
- Direct surveillance of epidemic or pandemic outbreaks.

Profile Needed:

- B.Pharm/M. Pharm.

4.8.2   Medical Transcription

Job Description:

- Able to deliver 500-600 lines, maintain 95 - 98% accuracy.
- Work minimum of 8-9 hours/day.
- TAT (Turn around Time) is of minimal duration as they are STAT (Sooner Than Already There).
- Must adhere HIPAA (*Health Insurance Portability and Accountability*) regulatory guidelines.

Profile Needed:

- B. Pharm, Graduate in Life Sciences.
- Should have good English Communication skills.
- Should have good experience in typing and MS office tools.

4.8.3   Clinical Data Management

Job Description:

- Work with complex computerized records systems and maintain security and integrity.
- Collect data from clinical trials.
- Sort information and then ensure its screening, grouping, summarizing, transcribing, coding.
- Consult with other employees to solve operational or data problems.
- Provide clerical duties such as data entry, transcription, coding, and collating searches.
- Prioritize work in line with project management decisions.
- Manage clinical trials through review, computerization, cleaning and auditing of clinical data and databases in compliance with standard operating procedures, client guidelines and regulatory agency guidelines.
- Validate clinical trial data to ensure consistency, integrity and accuracy based on project specific guidelines.
- Generate data retrievals and summaries.
- Query data inconsistencies and revise case report forms in compliance with standard operating procedures.
- Review case report forms for completeness and consistency.
- Implement strategy for data cleaning and the design and programming of clinical databases.
- Review and approve design, data review ground rules and database design according to standard operating procedures and protocol.

Profile Needed:

- A Bachelors/ Masters degree (preferably in Pharmacy, Health Sciences, Science or Clinical).

- A background in Medical Terminology, Pharmacology, Anatomy, and Physiology required for many tasks.

- A thorough understanding of clinical drug development process.

4.8.4 Pharmacovigilance

Pharmacovigilance/Medical device officer is responsible for instituting and maintaining the key aspects of medical device regulation. Additionally, the role involves collecting, monitoring, processing, and documenting of adverse reactions reported to all medical products.

The incumbent will provide guidance to health care providers to take responsibility for medication error detection, reporting, evaluation, and prevention and provide guidance to medical device suppliers to comply with regulatory requirements. Additional responsibilities include drafting regulatory policies, development of protocols, Standard Operating Procedures (SOPs) and all related duties to enable PV workflow and activities.

Job Description:

- Develop and implement appropriate controls for medical devices that are aligned to the Health Authority and policies.

- Provide scientific expertise and services to satisfy the expectations of the public, device users and hospital institutions and the medical device industry.

- Evaluate and regulate medical devices intended for use, with the objective of ensuring all medical devices sold meet the required safety, efficacy and quality standards, as devices and their performance according to their intended purpose within the scope of accepted regulatory practices.

- Review and approve devices for reimbursement by the relevant insurance companies.

- Routinely review, identify, investigate, alert, and where necessary, resolve safety issues for medical devices that could potentially affect the health and safety of patients.

- Assist with the development and creation of tools and programs to improve regulatory efficiencies.

Profile Needed:

Senior Manager- Pharmacovigilance Services

Qualification - MBBS / MD / MDS / M Pharm / B Pharm

- 7+ years of experience in global Pharmacovigilance in a reputed pharmaceutical company.

- Experience in Aggregate Reporting, Risk Evaluation & Management Strategies is required.
- Proficiency in Oracle AERS preferred.
- Excellent Communication Skills, Ability to manage & motivate team and a good understanding in Global PV Regulations.

Manager - Pharmacovigilance Service
Qualification- MBBS/ M Pharm / BDS / B Pharm

- 5+ years of experience in global Pharmacovigilance in a reputed pharmaceutical company.
- Experience in Aggregate Reporting, Risk Management and familiarity with Oracle AERS.

Assistant Manager - Pharmacovigilance Services
Qualification - MBBS / M Pharm / BDS / B Pharm

- 4+ years of experience in global Pharmacovigilance in a reputed pharmaceutical company.
- Experience in ICSR (individual case safety reports) Processing Reporting and PSUR (periodic safety update reports) / PADER (Periodic Adverse Drug Experience Report) Preparation and familiarity with Oracle AERS (Adverse Event Reporting System).

Call Centre Executive -Pharmacovigilance
Qualification: B Pharm / BDS / B. Sc (Nursing)

- 1-2 yrs of experience in call handling and with voice and accent training.
- Fresher with exceptional credentials.

Assistant Manager - Information Technology
Qualification - BE / MCA/ BCA/Any Graduate

- 4+ years experience in Oracle AERS Application Administration & TMS.
- Experience in handling Pharmacovigilance Data Base.

4.8.5 Prescription Data Base Maintenance

Job Description:

- Properly maintain the data of the prescription for smooth running of hospital.
- This gives an complete picture of what a patient may be receiving or a prescriber may be writing.
- The organization aims to achieve more consistent policy in promotion of adequate drug management and education of the medical community about treating within the bounds of professional practice and without fear of regulatory scrutiny.

Profile Needed:

- A Bachelors/ Masters degree (preferably in Pharmacy, Health Sciences, Science or Clinical).

4.8.6 Patient Care Advice

Patient care advice includes any role that enables patients and families to have direct input and influence on the policies, programs, and practices that affect the care and services that individuals and families receive.

Job Description:

- Meeting with 4 - 5 patients suffering from different ailments everyday (at the hospitals, clinics).
- Counseling and speaking to them for health outcomes management in person so that they understand the long-term implications of managed patient care.
- Collate health records related data from consenting patients.
- Meet the regular patients at regular intervals as advised.
- Capture details related to Adverse Drug Reactions reported by patient in pre-defined templates.
- Handling patient queries and providing response from pre-defined FAQs.
- Provide patient support by coordinating with pharmacists and stockists.
- Receive regular feedback from team managers and undergo program related training and on the job training on a regular basis.

Profile Needed:

- Qualifications: B. Pharm/ B. Sc (Microbiology, Biotechnology, Dietics, Nutrition) fresher – 2 years of experience.
- Fluent in English, Hindi and any one regional language.
- Good computer skills.
- Ability to work in a process driven/ structured environment.
- Empathy and willingness to listen and relate.

4.8.7 Quality Analyst

A **quality analyst** is responsible for applying the principles and practices of **quality** assurance in medical transcription.

Job Description:

- Must be a highly self motivated and qualified editor, Must transcribe and/or edit.
- Demonstrate ability to work in all work types and specialties.
- Demonstrate quality transcription work, consistently maintaining an accuracy score of 99% or high.

Profile Needed:

- **B. Pharm, Graduate in Life Sciences.**
- Minimum 3 years experience in Quality in Medical Transcription or 10 yrs of Medical Transcription experience.
- Auditing transcribed voice files.
- Good command over English and medical language.

4.8.8 Software Development

The software developer is responsible for developing all type of software used in Pharmaceutical sector.

Job Description:

- Candidate must have hands on experience and strong knowledge of ASP.NET (Active Server Pages Network Enabled Technologies) and C++.
- Must have hands on experience and strong knowledge on SQL (structured query language) server or Oracle.
- Experience in ASP.NET (Active Server Pages Network) 3.5 /4.0, Silver light applications, AJAX (*Asynchronous JavaScript and XML*) would be highly preferred.
- Should have complete SDLC (Software development lifecycle) experience on at least one project.
- Microsoft certification would be an added advantage.
- Develop software according to functional and technical design specifications and maintain a "common sense" approach that serves to recognize potential design gaps and provide insight into closing them.

Profile Needed:

- Must be a Graduate in any discipline.
- Candidates must have good aptitude and problem solving skills.
- Candidates should possess basic knowledge of OOPS (**Object-Oriented Programming System)**,HTML (*Hyper Text Markup Language*),CSS (*Cascading Style Sheets*), SQL (Software development lifecycle) server.

4.8.9 Medical Claims Processing

Insurance claims of patients in Clinics/Hospitals are managed by the medical claims processor. The claim processor analyzes and processes the insurance claim, and checks it thoroughly for validity.

Job Description:

- Validates the information of all medical claims from patients.

- Claims must be thoroughly reviewed to ensure that there is no missing or incomplete information.
- A processor must keep meticulous records of claims and follow up on lapsed cases.

Profile Needed:

- B. Pharm/ M. Pharm.
- Candidates having Certified Medical Reimbursement Specialist (CMRS) exam have the advantage.

4.8.10 SAS Programmer

Statistical Analysis System (SAS) is a software suite that can alter, manage and retrieve data from a variety of sources and perform statistical analysis on it.

Job Description:

- Programming, analyzing and evaluating clinical data using SAS.
- Ensure SAS programs adhere to specifications/Mock Shells and Program Oral Interpretation (POI) programming standards.
- Responsible for writing programming in order to generate tables and listings for clinical data on assigned projects for Production/Validation as assigned by Line Manager.
- Attend team meetings for assigned studies as appropriate.

Profile Needed:

- Bachelor's degree in a related field and 1-2+ years of experience.
- Pharmaceutical/clinical research experience required.
- Must be proficient with computer, MS Word, Excel and the Internet.
- Good SAS programming knowledge required.
- Thorough understanding of GCPs, CFR and ICH Guidelines.

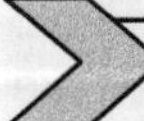 ## 4.9 Miscellaneous

Including the entire above sector few more fields are there where a Pharma student can create their career.

4.9.1 Community Pharmacy
Community Pharmacist in Middle East and Developed countries

4.9.2 Export & Import of Pharmaceuticals

4.9.3 Medical Writing

4.9.4 Pharmacist in Defense

4.9.5 Customs

4.9.6 Corporate sectors

4.9.7 Retail Pharmacy

4.9.1 Community Pharmacy

Community pharmacists are the health professionals most accessible to the public. They supply medicines in accordance with a prescription or, when legally permitted, sell them without a prescription. In addition to ensuring an accurate supply of appropriate products, their professional activities also cover counseling of patients at the time of dispensing of prescription and non-prescription drugs, drug information to health professionals, patients and the general public, and participation in health-promotion programmes. They maintain links with other health professionals in primary health care.

Job Description:

- Dispensing prescription medicines to the public.
- Ensuring that different treatments are compatible.
- Checking dosage and ensuring that medicines are correctly and safely supplied and labeled (pharmacists are legally responsible for any dispensing errors).
- Supervising the preparation of any medicines (not all are supplied ready made-up by the manufacturer).
- Keeping a register of controlled drugs for legal and stock control purposes.
- Liaising with doctors about prescriptions.
- Selling over-the-counter medicines.
- Counseling and advising the public on the treatment of minor ailments.
- Advising patients of any adverse side-effects of medicines or potential interactions with other medicines/treatments.
- Preparing rosette and cassette boxes, usually for the elderly but also for those with memory/learning difficulties, where tablets are placed in compartments for specified days of the week.
- Undertaking Medicine Use Reviews (MUR), an advanced service to help patients understand how their medicines work and why they have to take them.
- Providing a prescription intervention service.
- Managing a needle and syringe exchange.
- Measuring and fitting compression hosiery.
- Monitoring blood pressure and cholesterol levels.
- Offering a diabetes screening service.
- Arranging the delivery of prescription medicines to patients.
- Managing, supervising and training pharmacy support staff.
- Budgeting and financial management.

- Keeping up to date with current pharmacy practice, new drugs and their uses.

Profile Needed:

- Bachelor of Pharmacy.
- Certifications in different areas of pharmacy and an accredited residence program are a plus.
- However, certain personal abilities are all vital, such as communication abilities (both oral and written), deep knowledge on drugs, medical procedures and therapies, diagnosis and disease states, and pharmacokinetics.

Community Pharmacist in Middle East and Developed Countries

Job Description:

- Possible errors about the medication can be detected and reduced by pharmacists' interventions.
- The pharmacist is often the last member of the health care team to see the patient, before the patient starts using the drug. Additionally, pharmacists are accessible to patients, often seeing them on several occasions between routine physician visits. Therefore, it is the pharmacist's responsibility to ensure the safe and appropriate use of the medication by the patient.
- Information is as important as the appropriateness of the medicines themselves. The pharmacist must provide the necessary information and guidance to assure the patient's compliance in taking the medication properly.

Profile Needed:

- Bachelor of Pharmacy.
- Certifications in different areas of Pharmacy and an accredited residence program are a plus.
- However, certain personal abilities are all vital, such as communication abilities (both oral and written), deep knowledge on drugs, medical procedures and therapies, diagnosis and disease states, and pharmacokinetics.

4.9.2 Export & Import of Pharmaceuticals

A "licensed" or "registered" **importer** is one who has been granted a license or registration status for the purpose. Authorized **exporter means** an individual or company or similar legal entity **exporting** or seeking to **export** a **pharmaceutical** or veterinary product.

Job Description:

- An Import-Export Pharmacist / coordinator can work in various industries and often arranges communications between sales groups and national or international customers.
- Import-Export Pharmacists / coordinators are responsible for arranging shipments, preparing and confirming order approval, handling pricing information and releasing invoices.

Profile Needed:

- This position requires a bachelor's degree in Pharmacy and knowledge of standard regulations that go along with various domestic and international protocols.
- Courses in business including global business management, documentation and management.
- Understanding of domestic and world economy.
- Strong communication skills and basic computer skills.
- They must also manage their own team while also coordinating with other teams, dealing with customers.
- Since most Import-Export Pharmacists / coordinators interact with the International Business community, being fluent in a foreign language can be helpful.

4.9.3 Medical Writing

Medical Writing is an integral part of clinical research. **Medical Writers** work closely with their colleagues in the biostatistical, pharmacovigilance, project management, and clinical data management teams to deliver accurate, timely, and cost effective documents to the highest ethical and scientific standards.

Job Description:

- Under departmental supervision, the medical writer will research, create, edit, and coordinate the production of clinical documents associated with submissions to regulatory authorities including but not limited to: study protocols, model informed consents, interim and final clinical study reports and safety updates.
- The Medical Writer will also be responsible for the production of clinical study documentation associated with clinical trials that may not be included in a regulatory submission.
- Serve as the primary client contact, negotiating deliverable timelines, and resolving project related issues under departmental supervision. Project management of contractual and financial aspects may only be performed with the guidance of medical writing management.
- Serve as the Medical Writing representative on assigned project teams, providing proactive support to project leadership for planning efficient

work plans and timelines for medical writing deliverables, and medical writing input into other departmental deliverables.

- Identify any potential project challenges to departmental line management and project leader including changes in project plan, timeline or out of scope requests, and suggest possible resolution options.

- Provide medical editing review of draft and final documents prepared by other writers before internal or external distribution. This includes both copy editing and content review.

- Ensure document content and style adheres to FDA/EMA or other appropriate regulatory guidelines, and complies with departmental and corporate or client Standard Operating Procedures (SOPs) and style guidelines.

- Coordinate production and distribution of draft and final documents to project team and client. Ensure that all work is complete and of high quality prior to team distribution or shipment to client.

- Perform literature searches/reviews as necessary to obtain background information and training for development of documents.

- Review statistical analysis plans and mock statistical output to determine the appropriateness of content/format for clinical writing.

- Attend internal technical team and client team meetings as required.

- May provide guidance to less experienced departmental members.

- Supervise collection of materials by the Medical Writing Assistant or Associate Medical Writer for assembly of client deliverables and for filing appropriately in project files.

- May participate in departmental or inter departmental process improvement and training initiatives.

- May participate in development of formats, templates and general guidelines for clinical documentation and workflow procedures. Assist in the development of departmental Standard Operating Procedures (SOPs).

- Keep abreast of professional information and technology through workshops and conferences, and ensure the appropriate transfer of that information to the department.

Profile Needed:

- Bachelor's degree in Pharmacy, Life Sciences/Health Related Sciences or equivalent.

- Client focused approach to work.

- Willingness to work in a matrix environment and to value the importance of teamwork.

- Demonstrated understanding of the drug development process.

- Extensive clinical/scientific writing skills.
- Advanced word processing skills/familiarity with Word for Windows.
- Fluent in written and spoken English.

4.9.4 Pharmacist in Defense

Job Description:

- Checking prescriptions to ensure that there are no errors and are appropriate and safe for the individual patient.
- Providing advice on the dosage of medicines and the most appropriate form of medication, for example- tablet, injection, ointment or inhaler.
- Participating in ward rounds, taking patient drug histories and involvement in decision-making on appropriate treatments.
- Discussing treatments with patients relatives, community pharmacists and GPs.
- Ensuring medicines are stored appropriately and securely.
- Supervising the work of less experienced and less qualified staff.
- Answering questions about medicines from within the hospital, other hospitals and the general public.
- Keeping up to date with, and contributing to research and development.

Profile Needed:

- Degree or Diploma in Pharmacy from any recognized institution of the central or State Government for the period of Training in two years followed by an internship of which the practical training shall not be less than five hundred hour spread over a period of not less than three months.

4.9.5 Customs

Job Description:

- Checking prescriptions and medications of travelers at Airports.

Profile Needed:

- Degree or Diploma in Pharmacy.

4.9.6 Corporate Sectors

A Pharmacy graduate can join any corporate sector or bank as a Pharmacist.

Job Description

- All duties attached to Medical Clinic of the company as Pharmacist, including assisting in Clerical work, whenever necessary. Should be able to give first aid treatment independently in accident cases.

Profile Needed:
- Degree or Diploma in Pharmacy from any recognized institution.

4.9.7 Retail Pharmacy

A **pharmacy** in which drugs are sold to patients is called a Retail Pharmacy.

Job Description:
- Retail pharmacists dispense medications at drug stores.
- Assist with the development of new business and feedback acquisition through tele-calling & if needed counseling.
- Identify key trends and prospects.
- Provide additional support to sales team as necessary.
- Generate spreadsheets and reports using different kind of data.
- Need to work for 8 hours in day & ready to work in shifts.
- Need to prepare competitor analysis & create new project online.
- Need to generate business in specified period of time.

Profile Needed:
- Degree or Diploma in Pharmacy from any recognized institution of the Central or State Government.
- Strong communication skill.
- Organized with an ability to prioritize assignments.
- Creative, flexible & fast learner.
- Interest in non-profit management & community development.

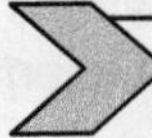

CHAPTER 5

Interview

5.1 Introduction

Interview is an important stage before final selection is made for any post. Only a few posts are filled without interview. Generally for each post seven to eight candidates are called for interview. It is the final hurdle which the candidate has to cross in order to get the job which he seeks.

The candidate has to remember that the interviewers are persons of wide knowledge & experience. They are able to judge the real character and worth of a candidate by his speech, expressions and self presentation. The Interviewers would not mind if the candidate is a little short of their expectations but he has to prove that he has a real aptitude for the job and can acquit himself creditably in it.

The candidate, therefore, has to give his best to the Interviewers. He/she must remember that the first impression is the last impression. In the very beginning he should impress the interviewer with his knowledge, intelligence and confidence. The candidate should not get perturbed when theinterviewer tries to screen him and play on his nerve. The candidate should try to retain his politeness, cheerfulness and patience to the end displaying his interest and sincerity in the interview all the time.

Some Fundamental Qualities

Confidence: If you have a strong will to win you will get the way. Lack of confidence arises out of your shortcomings. Try to know them and get rid of them. Try to be social and get opportunities to mix with different types of people with different habits. Do visit different places in order to get in touch with different types of people. This will go a long way in removing your shyness and nervousness. The more experience you gather in the above regards, the more confidence will develop.

Personality: Personality doesn't consist only of handsome features or a well built body. A winning personality is the keystone in the arch of success. Your personality is the greatest asset you will ever have. More than anything else it is your personality that will tilt the favor of the interviewers to your side. The definition of personality includes physique, appearance, intelligence, aptitudes and individual characteristic ways of conducting oneselfhimself in everyday situations. A positive personality is an asset which one must develop in order to be successful not only in the battle of interview but also in the complex struggle of life.

Expression: The way a candidate expresses his thoughts and ideas is very much responsible in deciding his fate at the interview. It is by your expression that you reveal your thinking power. Your answers should be short, precise, well worded and spoken in a clear and pleasing tone. Do not try to elaborate your answers unnecessarily. In every case every word should be clear. Your voice should be neither too loud nor too mild. Your face should wear a natural and cheerful smile and your tone should be very pleasing. Never try to enter in to an argument & if you are wrong admit it quickly without any hesitation.

Alertness: The candidate should be very much alert at the time of interview. He should take the minimum time in understanding the question of the interviewer. If you are unable to listen to the question then please ask again by saying "beg your pardon or sorry sir". If to every new question you say "beg your pardon or sorry sir", that shows your lack of attention

Manners: Your manner shows your status, breeding and background. When you enter the interview room you have to stand properly before the interviewers, your hands and head in the proper position. There is a term body language which speaks louder than the words you speak. Unnecessary movement of hand, head, shaking the legs while sitting, smattering , smiling or laughing without any valid reason, thumping the table to emphasize a point, sitting or standing in an abnormal way, all these things must be avoided. Constant practice can enable you to shake off these characteristics if unfortunately they have become a part of your personality.

Smartness: To catch the attention of the interviewer the candidate should be smartly dressed. The first impression created by the candidate on the interviewers will be by the dress. A smart dress does not necessarily mean a costly dress. First of all your clothes should be properly tailored and should fit you well. Your dress must be sober, simple and pleasing.

Hints for the Candidate:

1. The candidate should walk to his chair in the interviewer room quite normally.

2. Enter the room neither very hurriedly nor very slowly, you should walk in a normal pace.

3. Do not take your seat unless you are asking to do so.

4. Do not stand up when you are asked to answer a question. You should reply the questions sitting calmly in your seat.

5. You should not place your portfolio containing your testimonials etc. on the table.

6. Instead of keeping your hands below the table or on the table you should place them on the hands of your chair in a normal position.

7. Speak in a soft but very clear tone.

8. Do not get up & leave the room before you are asked to do so.

SOME DO'S AND DON'TS:

DO'S

1. Give your best to the interviewers.
2. Cover your weakness through the presentation of other achievements.
3. Remain unperturbed and composed and keep your interest throughout the interview.
4. First listen very attentively and carefully to the question put to you. Then answer it in a natural and normal way.
5. Adopt a pleasing manner of speech.
6. Develop your personality to suit the post for which you have applied.
7. Be prompt without being hasty, quick without being aggressive and civil without being cringing.
8. Establish a rapport with the interviewers.
9. Emit vivacity and enthusiasm from your looks and expressions.
10. Show pleasing and graceful manners, sufficient politeness and verve.
11. Gather adequate general knowledge before appearing in the interview.
12. Try to show your interest in the job and never give the impression that you are only casually appearing before the interviewers.

DON'TS

1. Do not appear nervous or shaky.
2. Do not try to elaborate your answer.
3. Do not interrupt the interviewer.
4. Do not enter into an argument with the interviewer.
5. Do not hesitate in answering questions.
6. Do not show ill manners.
7. Do not be aggressive.
8. Do not lose your presence of mind.
9. Do not try to bluff or confuse the interviewer.
10. Do not show your ignorance.
11. Do not talk more than what is needed.
12. Do not make unnecessary movements of any part of the body.

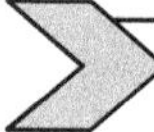

5.2 Task to do before Attending the Interview

- Thoroughly research the company.

  Check out its website, as well as its current status i.e. Financials, business issues and competitors on various sites like Yahoo Finance, Google Finance and Hoovers.com. Follow the company on social network site and see what people are saying.

- Take time to carefully review the job description or advertisement.

  Prepare short narratives of how and when you have done each thing that is mentioned. Be prepared to talk about obstacles you encountered and how you deal with them successfully. And by all means, be prepared to talk about past achievements that you have attained which in any way relate to the work necessary for the job.

- Do an advanced people search on any social network site for current employees in the area of the company where you would be working, and review as many of their profiles as possible.

  When you are doing this, it is best to be in secrecy mode. Go into the Privacy and Settings menu, adjust what others see when you have looked at their profiles and click on the "You will be totally anonymous" button.

  Look for points that you have in common with individuals whose profiles you are reviewing. From this you may know about the kind of people the company likes to hire and the kind of achievements that are most valuable to the company. In short, seek out anything that will give you a tip off about the kind of people that the company likes to hire and the kind of achievements that are most valuable to the company.

  Prepare as well to subtly mention any points of commonality that you share, whether it is a past city, company, school, etc.

- Prepare to ask intelligent questions.

  Never ask a question that you would know the answer to if you had done your homework. Instead, show your engagement and background by asking, "Do you do X this way or that way?" Show your desire to go above and beyond by asking, "What are the most important contributions I can make in the first six months on the job?" And include this killer interview closing question.

  "If I'm hired and you give me a stellar review a year from now, what I would I have done to earn it?" If a job seeker approaches an interview with a perfect attitude matching to the job vacancy, then he or she can sharpen the points to be made in the interview and maximize the chances of hitting the bull's eye.

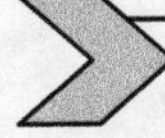

5.3 Questions Most Frequently Asked by HR / Other Experts About You

- Tell me about yourself OR introduce yourself.

  Talk about you your studies

  First of all I would like to thank you for giving an opportunity to introduce myself.

  My name is … (your name) I am from ……… (Area)

  I have completed my B. Pharm in this year from …… (Name of the Institute). I had completed my +2/ intermediate Sc. in … (e.g. 1999) from …… (Name of the Institute) & 10th / Matriculation in … (e.g. 1999) from …… (Name of the Institute)

  There are …. Members in my family

  My father's name is ……….. (Name of your father) & in Occupation he is a …. (Tell the occupation of your father)

  My mother's name is ……….. (Name of your mother) & in Occupation she is a …. (Tell the occupation of your mother)

  My hobbies is to ………………….. (Tell your hobbies)

  Tell your AIM/ Career Objective

- **Tell me something about your interest & activities.**

  Your answer should match the key aspects or job responsibilities of the job

- **What are your strengths and weaknesses?**

  Strengths: It's important to discuss attributes that will qualify you for the job. The best way to respond is to describe the skills. Here are few examples…

  My ability to work with different people with varying personalities I enjoy learning from everyone I meet.

  My strength is my ability to focus on the job at hand. I'm not easily distracted from the big picture.

  My organizational skills are my greatest strength. I'm capable of keeping many projects on track at the same time.

  I am a self motivated person, quick Learner & I will dedicate myself to my work.

  My time management skills are excellent and I'm organized, efficient, and take pride in excelling at my work.

  I pride myself on my customer service skills and my ability to resolve what could be difficult situations. Some of the strengths can be….

  Organizational and planning skills.

Perseverance / persistence / steadiness

Persuasive ability

Communication skills

Leadership ability

Stress tolerance

Ability to learn and apply new information and skills

Flexibility

Independence

Problem-solving

Creativity

Technical and professional knowledge

Reliability

Self-motivation

Initiative

Quick learner

Dedicated to my work

Proactive / complete task as it comes based on priority

The term **"Weakness"** isn't used in the answers - you always want to focus on the positive when interviewing. Always try to answer this type of questions in a positive or tricky way so that your weakness shows your strength. **For example,**

I've learned to make my perfectionism work to my advantage. I have become proficient at meeting deadlines, and with my attention to detail, I know my work is accurate. I used to leave assignments until the last minute, but with the workload of graduate school, I learned to schedule my time very effectively.

I used to like to work on one project to its completion before starting on another, but I've learned to balance work on several projects simultaneously, and I think it allows me to be more creative and effective.

I'm impatient with people who don't work at the same pace as me but I'm learning to manage this. I make sure that they have the right resources for the job; I follow up to see that they are on track and I step in and help when needed.

I've been reluctant to delegate. I have had to re-evaluate this as it was creating a big workload for me. I assign each person a specific, manageable task and then follow up to satisfy myself that it is being done properly, this seems to work well.

I can be a bit aggressive in reaching my goals.

At times *I can get too involved in other people's problems, trying to help them.*

Unable to sleep until work is completed.

**While telling your strength & weakness say 2 to 3 strengths & 1 to 2 weaknesses only.

- What attracts you to this organization/ setting/ position? Or why do you want to work in our Organization?
  Name of the organization, means you say for eg. The name Novartis stands for a lot.
  I need a platform to prove my skills & knowledge; your company is one of the best companies, so according to me it is the best platform for me.

- **What is the difference between confidence & over confidence?**

  Confidence makes a person feel released whereas over confidence always leaves you in doubt.

  Confidence makes a work process success but over confidence leads to failure.

- **What is the difference between hard work & smart work?**

  Hard work involves the total energy of body where as smart work involves little energy of mind.

  In hard work for output you have to put more effort but in smart work putting less effort you can get the output.

- **How do you define success & how do you measure up to your own definition?**

  Success means reach the target. If I will get the desired result then for me it is success.

  So according to me Success means to satisfy someone with your work.

- **How do you feel to work at night?**
  It's not a problem for me, I can manage. According to me we can work properly at night because there is less disturbance.

- **Can you work under pressure?**
  Yes, I can. Pressure helps me to do my best & my ability to adopt different situation. From this we also learn something.

- **Are you willing to relocate or travel?**
  Yes, I am ready to relocate or travel. I will be happy to interact with new people & learning about new culture.

- **What is your goal or where do you see yourself in five to ten years?**
  My short term goal is to get a job. My main goal is to work hard & be sincere, which place me in a good position in future and my organization will be proud of me.

- **What is most important to you: the money or the work?**
  The Work, in my opinion/ according to me I have to learn first.

- **What is the salary you are looking for in this position?**
  As per the company policy for fresher as a fresher I have to learn first.

- **Tell me about a project that you handled well and one in which you were not successful. What did you learn from each one?**
  It depends on you, always tell the interviewer about the project you handled well.

- **How will you rate yourself on a scale from one to ten?**
  As a fresher 6 or 7 (say any one).

- **Do you think company will accept you? If yes. 'Then why? Or How long would you work for the company if hire?**

  Yes, I can prove it by my work.

  Sir being a fresher I have no experience but as I assure you that in future I will be a **key asset** for your esteemed Organization.

  I think I am fortunate enough if you give me an opportunity. I will work for the company as long as the company needs my services & as long as I grow technically & economically along with the company.

- **Explain how would you be an asset of the company?**

  Being a fresher I will work hard & stick to the job assigned to me by putting my hundred percent effort, in this way I can be an asset of your company

- **Would you lie for our company?**

  Mostly No, because it creates more problems. And Yes, if by this my company would be benefited.

- **What was the toughest decision you ever had made?**

  My toughest decision is to take admission in B. Pharm after +2 Science. Inspired by few of my relatives I took admission in this Profession.

- **Tell me something about our company?**
  Name of the company

  Founded by & Year

  Products

  Manufacturing Plants & Marketing Strategy

  Few more details of the company

  e.g. **Sun Pharmaceuticals Ltd.**

  > **Founded:** 1983, Mumbai
  >
  > **Founder:** Dilip Shanghvi
  >
  > **CEO:** KalyanaSundaram Subramanian
  >
  > **Headquarters:** Mumbai, Maharashtra, India

Sun Pharmaceutical Industries Limited is an Indian global pharmaceutical company that manufactures and sells pharmaceutical formulations and active pharmaceuticals. Sun Pharmaceuticals was established by Mr. Dilip Shanghvi in 1983 in Kolkata with five products to treat psychiatry ailments, Cardiology products were introduced in 1987 followed by gastroenterology products in 1989. Today it is the largest chronic prescription company in India and a market leader in psychiatry, neurology, cardiology, orthopedics, ophthalmology, gastroenterology and nephrology. Some of the top brands of the company include Pantocid, Susten, Aztor, Gemer, Repace, Glucored, Strocit, Clopilet and Cardivas. Over 57% of Sun Pharma sales are from markets outside India, primarily in the US. Manufacturing facilities are across 23 locations, including the US, Canada, Brazil, Mexico and Israel. In the US, the company markets over 200 generics, with another 150 awaiting approval from the U.S. Food and Drug Administration (FDA).

- **Do you have any questions?**

Thank you sir, for this question. I think I am not the appropriate person to ask you any question. I have one question that is, what are the qualities which you would expect from the fresher like us or are my answers against your question matched. (you can also refer to 5.2)

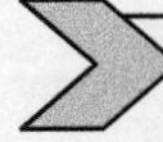

5.4   Questions Asked by Different Experts of Pharma Industry

- **What do you mean by A Production Trainee Chemist (PTC)?**

Production Trainee chemists use their knowledge of chemicals and their composition to assist with the production of various products such as drugs, cosmetics etc. They are employed in factories and work with production staff to ensure that production meets all deadlines as well as quality standards.

- **What are the job responsibilities of a PTC?**

Production chemists prepare directions for factory workers that include the proper ingredients, temperatures and mixing times for each step in the production process. They are also responsible for overseeing automated production methods to make sure that the desired product yield is achieved. Production chemists also analyze raw material samples and finished products to verify that they meet government and industry regulations. They must also record test results and provide feedback to the production staff so that production methods may be improved. Production chemists also work to develop new testing methods, which allow them to complete more work in a more efficient manner.

- **What qualities a PTC should have?**

Pleasing personality with leadership *qualities*, working knowledge to manage job duties, strong ethics as it is vital to keep data and sensitive information secured, strong attention to detail, quality oriented, strong oral and written communication skill, strong analytical ability, good organizational skills etc.

- **Why did you decide Pharmaceutical Production / QC / QA would be the right career for you?**

Being a Pharmacy graduate I chose this line because, this is the perfect platform for me.

- **What is the hierarchy of Pharmaceutical Production / QC / QA?**

Go to 4.1 of Chapter 4.

- **What is GMP, GLP & GCP?**

Good Manufacturing Practice (GMP) is the part of quality assurance which ensures that products are consistently produced and controlled to the quality standard appropriate to their intended use and as required by the marketing authorization or product specification.

GMP is concerned with both production and quality control.

The rules Governing Medicinal Products in the EU: Volume 4 – EU Guidelines to GMP Medicinal products for human and veterinary use.

Good Laboratory Practices (GLP) is a quality system concerned with the organizational process and the conditions under which non-clinical health and environmental safety studies are planned, performed, monitored, recorded, archived and reported.

GLPs are regulations published in the Code of Federal Regulations (21CFR part 58).

GLPs are not guidelines; they have the force of law.

Good Clinical Practice (GCP) is an international ethical and scientific quality standard for designing, conducting, recording, and reporting trials that involve the participation of human subjects.

Guideline for Good Clinical Practice – ICH Harmonization Tripartite Guideline.

- **What is Parenteral?**

Parenteral is para enteral or not enteral. It means the introduction of nutrition, a medication, or other substance into the body via a route other than the mouth or rectum, especially via infusion, injection or implantation.

Drugs are given by two general methods: enteral and parenteral administration. Enteral administration involves the esophagus, stomach, and small and large intestines (i.e., the gastrointestinal tract). Methods of administration include oral, sublingual (dissolving the drug under the tongue), and rectal. Parenteral routes do not involve the gastrointestinal tract, include intravenous (injection into a vein), subcutaneous (injection under the skin), intramuscular (injection into a muscle), inhalation (infusion through the lungs), and percutaneous (absorption through intact skin) and sublingual (dissolving the drug under the tongue).

- **What is Sterility?**

Sterility can be defined as the freedom from the presence of viable microorganisms.

- **What are the types of sterilization?**

There are four methods of sterilization that are used. Those methods are 1) Steam/ Moist heat (autoclave) sterilization, 2) Chemical vapor sterilization, 3) Dry heat sterilization, and 4) Ethylene oxide gas sterilization.

- **What is dry heat sterilization?**

The Dry-Heat sterilization process is accomplished by conduction; that is where heat is absorbed by the exterior surface of an item and then passed inward to the next layer. Eventually, the entire item reaches the proper temperature needed to achieve sterilization. The proper time and temperature for Dry-Heat sterilization is 160°C (320°F) for 2 hours or 170°C (340°F) for 1 hour instruments should be dry before sterilization since water will interfere with the process. Dry-heat destroys microorganisms by causing coagulation of proteins.

- **What is moist heat sterilization?**

Moist heat, as the name indicates, utilizes hot air that is heavily laden with water vapor and where this moisture plays the most important role in the process of sterilization.

Moist heat causes destruction of micro-organisms by denaturation of macromolecules, primarily proteins. Destruction of cells by lysis may also play a role. While "sterility" implies the destruction of free-living organisms which may grow within a sample, sterilization does not necessarily entail destruction of infectious matter.

- **What is Autoclave?**

Autoclaves are devices that are designed to sterilize a variety of lab equipment and media for growing lab cultures. Autoclaves are also used to sterilize medical tools and piercing equipments. Their primary purpose is to make these items free from bacterial contamination by using a combination of high heat and high pressure.

- **What is Validation?**

In the pharmaceutical, medical device, food, blood establishments, tissue establishments, and clinical trials industries, **validation** is the documented act of demonstrating that a procedure, process, and activity will consistently lead to the expected results. It often includes the qualification of systems and equipment. It is a requirement for good manufacturing practices and other regulatory requirements.

- **What is clean room?**

A clean room is that which is maintained free of contaminants such as dust or bacteria. Clean rooms are used in laboratory work.

- **What are the types of aseptic condition?**

An Aseptic technique is a set of scrupulous specific practices or rules and procedures under controlled conditions so as to prohibit or minimize contamination of objects (specimens, work surfaces, equipment) in the Microbiology laboratory, of surgical or process room.

Types of aseptic techniques are as follows:

Flaming

Use of lab coats, hand gloves and mask

Radiation

Chemical disinfectants (liquid or gases)

Chemical antiseptics

Use of Laminar flow cabinet

- **What is Standard Operating Procedure (SOP)?**

Standard Operating Procedure is a document which describes the regularly recurring operations relevant to the quality of the investigation. The purpose of a Standard Operating Procedure (SOP) is to carry out the operations correctly and always in the same manner. A Standard Operating Procedure (SOP) should be available at the place where the work is done.

- **What is a Validation Summary Report?**

Validation Summary Reports provide an overview of the entire validation project. When regulatory auditors review validation projects, they typically begin by reviewing the summary report. The validation summary report should include A description of the validation project, all test cases performed including those test cases passed without issue, all deviations reported including how those deviations were resolved.

- **What is a Validation plan?**

Validation Plans define the scope and goals of a validation project. Validation plans are written before a validation project and are specific to a single validation project. Validation Plans can include:

Deliverables (Documents) to be generated during the validation process
Resources/Departments/Personnel to participate in the validation project
Time-Line for completing the validation project.

- **What is the role of QC?**

  Quality control (QC) is a procedure or set of procedures intended to ensure that a manufactured product or performed service adheres to a defined set of quality criteria or meets the requirements of the client or customer. QC is similar to, but not identical with, quality assurance (QA).

- **What is the role of QA?**

  QA is defined as a procedure or set of procedures intended to ensure that a product or service under development (before work is complete, as opposed to afterwards) meets specified requirements. QA is sometimes expressed together with QC as a single expression, quality assurance and control (QA/QC).

- **Difference between QA & QC?**

Quality Assurance	Quality Control
Quality **Assurance** makes sure you are doing the right things, the right way.	Quality **Control** makes sure the results of what you've done are what you expected.
QA aims to prevent defects with a focus on the process used to make the product. It is a **proactive** quality process.	QC aims to identify (and correct) defects in the finished product. Quality control, therefore, is a **reactive** process.
The goal of QA is to improve development and test processes so that defects do not arise when the product is being developed.	The goal of QC is to identify defects after a product is developed and before it's released.
QA is process oriented. Quality needs to be assured at every step of the process	QC is product oriented. Quality is verified after the product is developed
QA includes prevention of quality problems through planned and systematic activities including documentation.	QC includes the activities or techniques used to achieve and maintain the product quality, process and service.
An overall management plan to guarantee the standard of the drug.	A series of analytical measurements used to assess the quality of the drug.
Quality Assurance is the process or set of processes used to measure and assure the quality of a product.	Quality Control is the process of meeting products and services to consumer expectations.

- **What is IPQA & CQA?**

  In Process Quality Assurance & Corporate Quality Assurance.

- **What are the different dosage forms?**

  Oral

  Pill, i.e. tablet or capsule.

Specialty tablet like buccal, sub-lingual, or orally-disintegrating

Thin film (e.g., Listerine Pocketpacks)

Liquid solution or suspension (e.g., drink or syrup)

Powder or liquid or solid crystals

Natural or herbal plant, seed, or food of sorts (e.g., marijuana such as that found in "special brownies")

Pastes (e.g., Colgate brand toothpaste)

Inhalational

Aerosol

Inhaler

Nebulizer

Smoking

Vaporizer

Parenteral

Intra Dermal (ID)

Intra Muscular (IM)

Intra Osseous (IO)

Intra Peritoneal (IP)

Intra Venous (IV)

Subcutaneous (SC)

Intra Thecal (IT) Injection into the spinal column

Sublingual

Topical

Cream, gel, liniment or balm, lotion, or ointment, etc.

Ear drops (otic)

Eye drops (ophthalmic)

Skin patch (transdermal)

Vaginal rings

Suppository

Vaginal (e.g., douche, pessary, etc.)

rectal

- **What are the excepients used in tablets?**

Antiadherents:	e.g. Magnesium stearate
Binders:	e.g. Sucrose, lactose
Coatings:	e.g. Synthetic polymers, shellac
Disintegrants:	e.g. Sodium starch glycolate.

Fillers:	e.g. Dibasic calcium phosphate
Flavours:	e.g. Mint, cherry
Colours:	e.g. Amaranth
Lubricants:	e.g. Vegetable stearin, magnesium stearate
Glidants:	e.g. Fumed silica, talc
Sorbents:	e.g. Fatty acids, waxes, shellac
Preservatives:	e.g. Amino acids cysteine and methionine
Sweeteners:	e.g. Sugar

- **What is Tablet?**

A *tablet* is a pharmaceutical dosage form. *Tablets* may be *defined* as the solid unit dosage form of medicament or medicaments with or without suitable diluents and prepared either by molding or by compression.

- **What is Capsule?**

A solid dosage form in which a drug is enclosed in a hard or soft soluble container or "shell" of a suitable form of gelatin.

- **Name& explain at least five type of problem in tablet defects.**

The defects related to Tabletting Process

Capping: It is partial or complete separation of the top or bottom of tablet due to air-entrapment in the granular material.

Lamination: It is separation of tablet into two or more layers due to air-entrapment in the granular material.

Cracking: It is due to rapid expansion of tablets when deep concave punches are used.

The defects related to Excipient

Chipping: It is due to very dry granules.

Sticking: It is the adhesion of granulation material to the die wall.

Picking: It is the removal of material from the surface of tablet and its adherance to the face of punch.

- **Note different units of tablet hardness.**

Kilogram (kg) – The kilogram is recognized by the SI system as the primary unit of mass.

Newton (N) – The Newton is the SI unit of force; the standard for tablet hardness testing. 9.807 Newtons = 1 kilogram.

Pound (lb) – Technically a unit of mass but can also be used for force and should be written as pound force or lbf in this case. Sometimes used for tablet strength testing in North America, but it is not an SI unit. 1 kilogram = 2.204 pounds.

Kilopond (kp) – Not to be confused with a pound. A unit of force also called a kilogram of force. Still used today in some applications, but not recognized by the SI system. 1 kilopond = 1 kgf.

Strong-Cobb (SC) – An ad hoc unit of force which is a legacy of one of the first tablet hardness testing machines. Although the SC is arbitrary, it was recognized as the international standard from the 1950s to the 1980s. 1 Strong-Cobb represented roughly 0.7 kilogram of force or about 7 Newton's. Although the Strong-Cobb unit is arbitrarily based on the dial reading of a hardness tester, it became an international standard for tablet hardness in the 1950s until it was superseded by testers using SI units in the 1980s. The Strong-Cobb is a unit with a very unusual name for a unit of measurement since it is named after the company, Strong-Cobb Inc. The inventor of the hardness tester was Robert Albrecht, the plant engineer for the Strong-Cobb Company. He sold the patent to the company for $1.00.

- **Relationship of Capsule Shell size vs. fill weight.**

Empty Hard Gelatin Capsule Physical Specifications				
Size	Outer Diameter (mm)	Height or Locked Length(mm)	Actual Volume (ml)	Typical Fill Weights (mg) 0.70 Powder Density
000	9.97	26.14	1.37	960
00	8.53	23.30	0.95	665
0	7.65	21.7	0.68	475
1	6.91	19.4	0.50	350
2	6.35	18.0	0.37	260
3	5.82	15.9	0.30	210
4	5.31	14.30	0.21	145
5	4.91	11.10	0.13	90

- **List of common hardness testers**

  Monsanto tester.

  Strong-Cobb tester.

  Pfizer tester.

  Erweka tester.

  Dr. Schleuniger Pharmatron tester.

- **What is Stability study?**

  It is the capacity or the capability of a particular formulation in a specific container to remain within a particular chemical, microbiological, therapeutically and toxicological specifications.

USP defines stability of pharmaceutical product as, "extent to which a product retains with in specified limits and throughout its period of storage and use (i.e. shelf life).

- **What is Control Release, Immediate Release, Sustain Release, Delayed Release, Extended Release Formulation**

Control Release: Controlled drug delivery is one which delivers the drug at a predetermined rate, for locally or systemically, for a specified period of time.

Immediate Release: Immediate release tablets are those which disintegrate rapidly and get dissolved to release the medicaments. Immediate release may be provided by an appropriate pharmaceutically acceptable diluents or carrier which does not prolong, to an appreciable extent, the rate of drug release and/or absorption.

Sustain Release: **dosage forms** are designed to release a drug at a predetermined rate in order to maintain a constant drug concentration for a specific period of time with minimum side effects.

Delayed Release: A dosage form that releases a discrete portion or portions of drug at a particular time. An initial portion may be released promptly after administration. Enteric-coated dosage forms are common delayed-release products.

Extended Release: A dosage form that allows at least a twofold reduction in dosage frequency as compared to that drug presented as an immediate-release (conventional) dosage form.

- **Principles of HPLC, UV, IR, FTIR, Karl Fischer**

High Performance Liquid Chromatography (HPLC):

High performance liquid chromatography is now one of the most powerful tools in analytical chemistry. It has the ability to separate, identify, and quantify the compounds that are present in any sample that can be dissolved in a liquid. Today, compounds in trace concentrations as low as *parts per trillion* [ppt] may easily be identified. HPLC can be, and has been, applied to just about any sample, such as pharmaceuticals, food, nutraceuticals, cosmetics, environmental matrices, forensic samples, and industrial chemicals.

HPLC has been used for medical (e.g. detecting vitamin D levels in blood serum), legal (e.g. detecting performance enhancement drugs in urine), research (e.g. separating the components of a complex biological sample, or of similar synthetic chemicals from each other), and manufacturing (e.g. during the production process of pharmaceutical and biological products) purposes.

Principle HPLC:

High performance liquid chromatography (HPLC) is basically a highly improved form of column liquid chromatography. Instead of a solvent being allowed to drip through a column under gravity, it is forced through under high pressures of up to 400 atmospheres. That makes it much faster. All chromatographic separations, including HPLC operate under the same basic principle; separation of a sample into its constituent parts because of the difference in the relative affinities of different molecules for the mobile phase and the stationary phase used in the separation.

Ultraviolet–visible spectroscopy or ultraviolet-visible spectrophotometry (UV-Vis or UV/Vis) refers to absorption spectroscopy or reflectance spectroscopy in the ultraviolet-visible spectral region.

Principle:

Molecules containing π-electrons or non-bonding electrons (n-electrons) can absorb the energy in the form of ultraviolet or visible light to excite these electrons to higher anti-bonding molecular orbitals. The more easily excited the electrons (i.e. lower energy gap between the HOMO and the LUMO), the longer the wavelength of light it can absorb.

Beer-Lambert law:

The **Beer-Lambert law (or Beer's law)** is the linear relationship between absorbance and concentration of an absorbing species. The general Beer-Lambert law is usually written as:

$$A = a(\lambda) * b * c$$

Where A is the measured absorbance, $a(\lambda)$ is a wavelength-dependent absorptivity coefficient, **b** is the path length, and **c** is the analyte concentration. When working in concentration units of molarity, the *Beer-Lambert law* is written as: $A = \varepsilon * b * c$

Where ε is the wavelength-dependent molar absorptivity coefficient with units of M^{-1} cm^{-1}.

Infrared spectroscopy (IR spectroscopy) is the spectroscopy that deals with the infrared region of the electromagnetic spectrum that is light with a longer wavelength and lower frequency than visible light. It covers a range of techniques, mostly based on absorption spectroscopy. As with all spectroscopic techniques, it can be used to identify and study chemicals. For a given sample which may be solid, liquid, or gaseous, the method or technique of infrared spectroscopy uses an instrument called an **infrared spectrometer** (or spectrophotometer) to produce an infrared spectrum. A basic IR spectrum is essentially a graph of infrared light absorbance (or transmittance) on the vertical axis vs. frequency or wavelength on the horizontal axis. Typical units of frequency used in IR spectra are reciprocal centimeters (sometimes called wave numbers), with the symbol cm^{-1}. Units of IR wavelength are commonly given in micrometers (formerly called "microns"), symbol μm, which are related to wave numbers in a reciprocal way. A common laboratory instrument that uses this technique is a **Fourier transform infrared** (FTIR) spectrometer.

Principle:

Molecules are made up of atoms linked by chemical bonds. The movement of atoms and chemical bonds are like spring and balls (vibration). This characteristic of vibration called natural frequency of vibration. When energy in the form of infrared is applied then it causes the vibration between the atoms of the molecules when,

Applied infrared frequency = Natural Frequency of vibration

Then, absorption of IR radiation takes place and a peak is observed. Different functional groups absorb characteristic frequencies of IR radiation. Hence gives the characteristic peak value. Therefore, IR Spectrum of a chemical substance is a finger print of a molecule for its identification.

The infrared portion of the electromagnetic spectrum is usually divided into three regions; the near-, mid- and far- infrared, named for their relation to the visible spectrum. The higher-energy near-IR, approximately 14000–4000 cm^{-1} (0.8–2.5 µm wavelength) can excite overtone or harmonic vibrations. The mid-infrared, approximately 4000–400 cm^{-1} (2.5–25 µm) may be used to study the fundamental vibrations and associated rotational-vibrational structure. The far-infrared, approximately 400–10 cm^{-1} (25–1000 µm), lying adjacent to the microwave region, has low energy and may be used for rotational spectroscopy.

Karl Fischer titration is a classic titration method in analytical chemistry that uses coulometric or volumetric titration to determine trace amounts of water in a sample. It was invented in 1935 by the German chemist Karl Fischer.

- **What is a PQ Document?**

Performance Qualifications are a collection of test cases used to verify that a system performs as expected under simulated real-world conditions. The performance qualification tests requirements were defined in the User Requirement Specification (or possibly the Functional Requirements). Due to the nature of performance qualifications, these tests are sometime conducted with power users as the system is being released.

- **What is an OQ Document?**

Operational Qualifications are a collection of test cases used to verify the proper functioning of a system. The operational qualification tests requirements were defined in the Functional Requirements. Operational Qualifications are usually performed before the system is released for use.

- **What is an IQ document?**

Installation Qualifications are a collection of test cases used to verify the proper installation of a System. The requirement to properly install the system was defined in the Design Specification. Installation Qualifications must be performed before completing Operational Qualification or Performance Qualification.

- **What is 21 CFR part 11?**

Title 21 CFR Part 11 of the Code of Federal Regulations deals with the Food and Drug Administration (FDA) guidelines on electronic records and electronic signatures in the United States. Part 11, as it is commonly called, defines the criteria under which electronic records and electronic signatures are considered to be trustworthy, reliable and equivalent to paper records.

- **What is a Change Control?**

Change Control is a general term describing the process of managing how changes are introduced into a controlled System. In validation, this means how changes are made to the validated system. Change control is required to demonstrate to regulatory authorities that validated systems remain under control after system changes. Change Control systems are a favorite target of regulatory auditors because they vividly demonstrate an organization capacity to control its systems.

- **Why water for pharmaceutical use is always kept in close loop in continuous circulation?**

Water is a best medium for growth of many microorganisms. Microorganisms tend to settle on a surface if water is allowed to stand in a stagnant position for few hours, these settled microorganism form a film over the surface of vessel and piping, such film formed by microorganisms is also called as biofilm. Biofilms are very difficult of remove, once a biofilm is formed at a particular point then that point may form a biofilm very easily again even after cleaning as seed from this point may not be completely get removed effectively.

Biofilms then can become a source of microbial contaminations; therefore purified water after collection in a distribution system is always kept in a closed loop in a continuous circulation.

A continuous circulation is also not enough at some points, therefore it is aided with high temperature range from 65 °C to 80°C, a minimum temperature of 65 °C is considered a self sanitizing, but better assurance is obtained with a temperature of 80°C. Purified water collected should be stored in a stainless steel vessel which must facilitate distribution to the point of use in a closed loop of continuous circulation. Tank should be made of corrosion free material of construction, and must facilitate sanitization and easy cleaning.

- **Water for pharmaceutical use shall be free of cations, anions and other impurities why?**

  Water for pharmaceutical use must be free from inorganic as well as organic impurities, minerals, and heavy metals. Some impurities like calcium, magnesium, ferrous etc are responsible for degradation of drug molecule. Many cations like ferrous and calcium magnesium act as catalysts in degradation reaction of drug molecule, Anions like chloride are highly active as they participate in nucleophylic substitution reactions, where in they break a double bond between -C=C- in to a single bond as $Cl-CH-CH_2$-. This is why we observe that color dyes tend to fade in presence of chlorine as most of the dyes used are diazo compounds which has enough places for nucleophylic substitution reactions, which is also a reason why stability of drug is drastically affected in presence of cations and anions from mineral origin present in water.

- **Water for pharmaceutical use shall be free from heavy metals, why?**

  Heavy metals like lead and arsenic are highly cumulative neurotoxic metals. Heavy metals are not eliminated out of our body easily like other drugs and molecules but heavy metals bind with proteins and tend to get accumulated in fatty tissues. Nerve tissue is most likely to get damaged by heavy metals. So water must be free from heavy metals.

- **What is stress testing?**

  Stress testing is likely to be carried out on a single batch of the drug substance. The testing should include the effect of temperatures (in 10°C increments (e.g., 50°C, 60°C) above that for accelerated testing), humidity (e.g., 75 percent relative humidity or greater) where appropriate, oxidation and photolysis on the drug substance. The testing should also evaluate the susceptibility of the drug substance to hydrolysis across a wide range of pH values when in solution or suspension.

- **According to WHO guidelines what is the storage condition of climatic zone IVa and zone IVb?**

  Zone IV a: 30°C and 65% RH (hot and humid countries).

  Zone IV b: 30°C and 75% RH (hot and very humid countries).

- **What is the purpose of stress testing in stability studies?**

  Stress testing of the drug substance can help to identify the likely degradation products, which can in turn help establish the degradation pathways and the intrinsic stability of the molecule and validate the stability indicating power of the analytical procedures used. The nature of the stress testing will depend on the individual drug substance and the type of drug product involved.

- **What is the formula for calculating number of air changes in an area?**

  Number of air changes/hour in an area is

  $$\frac{\text{Total room airflow in CFM} \times 60}{\text{Total volume of room in cubic feet}}$$

  For calculating Total Room Airflow in CFM, first calculate air flow of individual filter. Formula is given below.

  Air flow (in cfm) = Avg. air velocity in feet/Minute x Effective area of filter

  Then find Total air flow. Formula is

  Total Air flow = Sum of air flow of individual filter.

  Air flow Velocity can be measured with the help of Anemometer.

- **What are the recommended bio burden limits of purified water & WFI?**

  Purified water has a recommended bio burden limit of 100 CFU/ml, and water for injection (WFI) has a recommended bio burden limit of 10 CFU/100 mL.

- **Brief about ICH stabilty guidelines?**

  Q1A- Stability testing of new drug substance & products.

  Q1B- Photo stability testing of new drug substances & products.

  Q1C-Stability testing of new dosage forms.

  Q1D-Bracketing & Matrix designs for testing of new drug substances and products.

  Q1E-Evaluation of stability data.

  Q1F-Stability data package for registration applications in climatic zone III & IV (Withdrawn).

- **What are significant changes in stability testing?**

  A 5% change in assay for initial value.

  Any degradation products exceed its acceptance criterion.

  Failure to meet acceptance criterion for appearance, physical attributes and functionality test.

  Failure to meet acceptance criteria for dissolution of 12 units.

- **If leak test fail during in process checks what needs to be done?**

  Immediately stop packing process and check for sealing temperature.

  Verify for any possible changes like foil width, knurling etc.

  Check & quarantine the isolated quantity of packed goods from last passed in process.

  Collect random samples & do retest.

  Blisters from the leak test passed containers shall allow going further and rest must be deblistered / defoiled accordingly.

- **How many Tablets shall be taken for checking friability?**

For tablets with unit mass equal or less than 650 mg, take sample of whole tablets corresponding to 6.5g. For tablets with unit mass more than 650mg; take a sample of 10 whole tablets.

- **What is the formula for calculating weight loss during friability test?**

$$\% \text{ Weight loss} = \frac{\text{Initial weight} - \text{Final weight} \times 100}{\text{Initial weight}}$$

- **What is the pass or fail criteria for friability test?**

Generally the test is run for once. If any cracked, cleaved or broken tablets present in the tablet sample after tumbling, the tablets fails the test. If the results are doubtful, or weight loss is greater than the targeted value, the test should be repeated twice and the mean of the three tests determined. A mean weight loss from the three samples of not more than 1.0% is considered acceptable for most of the products.

- **What is the standard number of rotations used for friability test?**

100 rotations

- **What is the fall height of the tablets in the friabilator during friability testing?**

6 inches

- **Why do we check hardness during in process checks?**

To determine the need of the pressure adjustments on the tablet machine. Hardness can affect the disintegration time. If tablet is too hard, it may not disintegrate in the required period of time. And if tablet is too soft it will not withstand handling and subsequent processing such as coating, packing etc.

- **What are the factors which influence tablet hardness?**

Compression force

Binder quantity (More binder more hardness)

Moisture content

- **Which type of tablets is exempted from Disintegration testing?**

Chewable Tablets

- **Which capsule is bigger in size - size '0' or size '1'?**

'0' size

- **What is the recommended temperature for checking DT of a dispersible tablet?**

$25 \pm 1^{0}\text{C}$ **(IP)** & $15 - 25^{0}\text{C}$ **(BP)**

- **What is mesh aperture of DT apparatus?**

1.8 -2.2mm (#10)

- **What is the pass / fail criteria for disintegration test?**

  If one or two tablets/capsules out of 6 fail to disintegrate completely, repeat the test on another 12 additional dosage units. The requirement is meeting if not fewer than 16 out of 18 tablets/capsules tested are disintegrated completely.

- **What are the recommended storage conditions for empty hard gelatin capsules?**

  15 - 25^{0}C & 35 -55% RH

- **Which method is employed for checking "Uniformity of dosage unit"?**

  Content uniformity

  Weight Variation

  Weight variation is applicable for following dosage forms; hard gelatin capsules, uncoated or film coated tablets, containing 25mg or more of a drug substance comprising 25% or more by weight of dosage unit

- **What is the recommended upward and downward movement frequency of a basket-rack assembly in a DT apparatus?**

  28 – 32 cycles per minute.

- **When performing the 'uniformity of weight' of the dosage unit, how many tablet/capsule can deviate the established limit?**

  Not more than two of the individual weights can deviate from the average weight by more than the percentage given in the pharmacopeia, and none can deviate more than twice that percentage.

Weight Variation limits for Tablets

IP/BP	Limit	USP
80 mg or less	10%	130mg or less
More than 80mg or Less than 250mg	7.5%	130mg to 324mg
250mg or more	5%	More than 324mg

Weight Variation limits for Capsules

IP	Limit
Less than 300mg	10%
300mg or more	7.5%

- **What needs to be checked during in process QA checks?**

  Environmental Monitoring

  Measured values obtained from the process equipment (ex: temperature, RPM etc.)

  Measured values obtained from persons (ex: timings, entries etc.)

  Process attributes (Ex: weight, hardness, friability etc.)

- **What precautions shall be taken while collecting in process samples?**

  While collecting in process samples, avoid contamination of the product being sampled (Don't collect samples with bare hands) & avoid contamination of sample taken.

- **In a tablet manufacturing facility 'positive' pressure is maintained in** processing area or service corridors?

  In tablet manufacturing facilities, pressure gradients are maintained to avoid cross contamination of products through air. Usually processing areas are maintained under positive pressure with respect to service corridors.

- **If sticking observed during tablet compression what may be the probable reason for the same?**

  If the granules are not dried properly sticking can occur.

  Too little or improper lubrication can also leads to sticking.

  Sticking can occur because of too much binder or hygroscopic granules.

- **What checks shall be carried out, while calibrating DT apparatus?**

  While calibrating DT apparatus, following checks shall be performed.

  Number of strokes per minute (Limit: 29-32 cycles/min)

  Temperature by probe & standard thermometer (Limit: $37 \pm 1\ ^{\circ}C$).

  Distance travelled by basket (Limit: 53 -57mm)

- **What is in process checks?**

  In process checks are checks performed during an activity, In order to monitor and, if necessary, to adjust the process to ensure that product confirms to its specification.

- **What is the difference between disintegration and dissolution?**

  Disintegration is a disaggregation process, in which an oral dosage form falls apart in to smaller aggregates. Disintegration time is the 'break up' time of a solid dosage form.

  Dissolution is a process by which solid substance enters in the solvent to yield a solution. It is controlled by the affinity between the solid substance and the solvent.

  In other words disintegration is a subset of dissolution.

- **Why do we calibrate a qualified equipment/instrument on definite intervals?**

  An equipment or instrument can 'drift' out of accuracy between the time of qualification and actual use. So it is recommended to calibrate and recalibrate the measuring devices and instruments on predetermined time intervals, to gain confidence on the accuracy of the data.

- **Why do we consider three consecutive runs/batches for process validation? Why not two or four?**

  The number of batches produced in the validation exercise should be sufficient to allow the normal extent of variation and trends to be established and to provide sufficient data for evaluation and reproducibility.

  First batch quality is accidental (co-incidental),

  Second batch quality is regular (accidental),

  Third batch quality is validation (confirmation).

  In 2 batches we cannot assure the reproducibility of data,4 batches can be taken but the time and cost are involved.

- **Explain about revalidation criteria of AHU system?**

  AHU system shall be revalidated periodically as mentioned in the regulatory standards. AHU shall be revalidated in following cases also.

  When basic design of AHU is changed,

  When clean room volume is changed,

  When new equipment is installed

  When a construction is carried out, that calls for reconstruction of AHU system.

- **What needs to be checked during AHU validation?**

  During AHU validation, following tests shall be carried out:

  Filter efficiency test,

  Air velocity & number of air changes,

  Air flow pattern (visualization)

  Differential pressure, temperature and RH

  Static condition area qualification

  Dynamic condition qualification

  Non-viable count

  Microbial monitoring

  Area recovery and power failure study

- **Position of oblong tablets to be placed in hardness tester to determine the hardness- Lengthwise / widthwise?**

  Position of oblong tablets should be length wise because the probability of breakage is more in this position.

- **Explain in detail about qualification of pharmaceutical water system?**

  Qualification of pharmaceutical water system involves three phases

Phase -1

A test period of 2-4 weeks should be spent for monitoring the system intensively. During this period the system should operate continuously without failure or performance deviation. Water cannot be used for pharmaceutical manufacturing in this phase. The following should be included in testing approach.

Under take chemical & microbiological testing in accordance with a defined plan.

Sample incoming feed water daily to verify its quality.

Sample each step of purification process daily.

Sample each point of use daily.

Develop appropriate operating ranges.

Demonstrate production and delivery of product water of required quantity and quality.

Use and refine the SOP's for operation, maintenance, sanitization and trouble shooting.

Verify provisional alert and action levels.

Develop and refine test failure procedure.

Phase -2

A further test period of 2-4 weeks. Sampling scheme will be same as Phase – 1.Water can be used for manufacturing process in this phase.

Approach should also demonstrate

- Consistent operation within established ranges.
- Consistent production & delivery of water of required quality and quantity.

Phase -3

Phase 3 runs for one year after satisfactory completion of phase-2. Water can be used for manufacturing process during this process.

- **What is the difference between calibration and Validation?**

Calibration is a demonstration that, a particular instrument or device produces results within specified limits by comparisons with those produced by a reference or traceable standard over an appropriate range of measurements.

Whereas Validation is a documented program that provides high degree of assurance that a specific process, method or system consistently produces a result meeting pre-determined acceptance criteria.

In calibration performance of an instrument or device is comparing against a reference standard. But in validation such reference standard is not used.

Calibration ensures that instrument or measuring devices producing accurate results. Whereas validation demonstrates that a process, equipment, method or system produces consistent results (in other words, it ensures that uniforms batches are produced).

- **What is bracketing & matrixing in stability testing?**

Both Matrixing & Bracketing are reduced stability testing designs.

Bracketing

The design of a stability schedule, such that only samples of extremes of certain design factors (ex: strength, package size) are tested at all time points as in full design. The designs assume that the stability of any intermediate level is represented by the stability of extremes tested.

Matrixing

The design of a stability schedule, such that a selected subset of possible samples for all factor combinations is tested at a specified time point. At a subsequent time point another subset of samples for all factor combination is tested. The design assumes that the stability of each subset samples tested represent the stability of all samples at a given time point.

Therefore a given time point other than initial & final ones not every batch on stability needs to be tested.

- **Briefly explain about ICH climatic zones for stability testing & long term storage conditions?**

ICH STABILITY ZONES

Zone	Type of Climate
Zone I	Temperate zone
Zone II	Mediterranean/subtropical zone
Zone III	Hot dry zone
Zone IVa	Hot humid/tropical zone
Zone IVb	ASEAN testing conditions hot/higher humidity

Long term Storage condition

Climatic Zone	Temperature	Humidity	Minimum Duration
Zone I	21°C ± 2°C	45% rH ± 5% rH	12 Months
Zone II	25°C ± 2°C	60% rH ± 5% rH	12 Months
Zone III	30°C ± 2°C	35% rH ± 5% rH	12 Months
Zone IV	30°C ± 2°C	65% rH ± 5% rH	12 Months
Zone IVb	30°C ± 2°C	75% rH ± 5% rH	12 Months
Refrigerated	5°C ± 3°C	No Humidity	12 Months
Frozen	-15°C ± 5°C	No Humidity	12 Months

- **What are the common variables in the manufacturing of tablets?**

  Particle size of the drug substance

  Bulk density of drug substance/excipients

  Powder load in granulator

  Amount & concentration of binder

  Mixer speed & mixing timings

  Granulation moisture content

  Milling conditions

  Lubricant blending times

  Tablet hardness

  Coating solution spray rate

- **Whether bracketing & validation concept can be applied in process validation?**

  Both Matrixing & Bracketing can be applied in validation studies.

  Matrixing

  Different strength of same product

  Different size of same equipment

  Bracketing - Evaluating extremes

  Largest and smallest fill volumes

  Fastest and slowest operating speeds

- **What is Normality?**

  It is defined as the number of gram equivalents per liter of solutions. Or It is a measure of concentration equal to gram equivalent weight per litre of Solution.

  Normality = Number of gram equivalents/ 1 L of Solution.

- **What is Molarity?**

  It is defined as the number of gram moles of solute per liter of solution.

  Molarity= Gram Moles of solute/ Liter of solution

- **What is Molality?**

  It is defined as the number of moles of solute per kilogram of solvent.

  Molality= Gram Moles of solute/ Kilogram of solvent

- **What is pH?**

  It is the –ve logarithm of hydrogen ion concentration in a solution.

  It is a figure expressing the acidity or alkalinity of a solution on a logarithimic scale on which 7 is neutral, lower values are more acid & higher values are more alkaline.

- **What is Conductivity?**

  It is defined as a material's ability to conduct electricity. Electric current can flow easily through a material with high conductivity. It is measured in Siemens per meter & is often represented using greek letter σ.

- **What is WFI?**

  WFI means Water for Injection.

  It is defined as the water that has been purified by distillation for the preparation of products for parenteral use.

- **What is UV?**

  UV light is an electromagnetic radiation with a wave length from 400 to 100 nm, shorter than that of visible light but longer than X rays.

- **What is IR?**

  Infrared radiation alone refers to energy in the region of the electromagnetic radiation spectrum at wave lengths longer than those of visible light, but shorter than those of radio waves.

- **What is HPLC?**

  HPLC stands for High Performance Liquid Chromatography.

  It is a technique in analytical chemistry used to separate, identify and quantify each component in a mixture.

- **What is GCMS?**

  GCMS stands for Gas chromatography–mass spectrometry.

  It is a technique for the analysis & quantization of organic volatile & semi volatile compounds. It is used to separate mixtures into individual components using a temperature controlled capillary column.

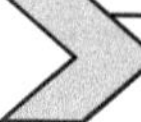

5.5 Questions for Medical Representatives

- **What do you mean by A Medical Representative**

  A person who represent the pros & cons of a medicine of his company in front of a Doctor.

- **What are the job responsibilities of a MR?**

  - To establish new molecule in the market by frequent discussion with doctors and at the same time to take care of existing products by giving growth.
  - To check the availability of products in the market by visiting chemists.
  - To take care of the payment structure which flows from the stockiest to company.
  - To have strict observation of the competitor activities and movement of their brands.
  - To maintain the good will of the company in the market.
  - To implement any strategy of the company.

- **What qualities a MR should have?**

  A MR should have the capacity to prioritize

  He should be strategy implementer.

  He always keeps his eye on the competitor activities.

  He should have decision making capacity.

  Lastly he should be a good planner.

- **Why did you decide pharmaceutical sales would be the right career for you?**

  Visiting Doctors in diurnal life is a great pleasure.

  I have been inspired by my Cousin Brother/ Brother in Law/ Friend/ Uncle.

  In this profession we can achieve a lot if we work properly.

  In this profession we are always spick & span.

- **How many hours you are able to work?**

  As we know that it is not an official job, so there is no time limitation.

  But I can manage

- **What do you think is the most challenging aspect of a pharmaceutical representative?**

  Well number one, I think it's probably getting quality time with the physician to impact prescribing behavior. Another challenge I think you would face is there are physicians that don't see representatives. You have to be creative in finding a way to gain access to them.

  The most difficult part is actually convincing a doctor to switch from a drug that she/he and their patients are quite comfortable with and present a new alternative, which may or may not be better. Of course, the target group of a pharmaceutical is quite different than a common salesman, but that is the least challenging aspect of a pharmaceutical sales representative.

- **What is the difference between marketing & sales?**

Marketing	Sales
It is a broader term than sales. It consist of public relations, branding, advertising & sales etc.	It is one part of activity of marketing. It is a narrower concept
It is creating the demand in the market	It is fulfilling the demand created by marketing
It is an indirect activity	It is a direct activity
It focuses on long term concerns	It is related with short term focus
It is related with educating & creating awareness of the product a service in the market on a huge scale (one to many)	It does those activities on a very short scale & most of the times one as one basis (One time)
It is pull strategy	It is push strategy
It shows how to reach to the customers	It is the ultimate result of marketing

- **Why did you think pharmaceutical sales job is better than other sales job?**

  A pharmaceutical sales representative has to sell medical drugs and other medical paraphernalia to doctors and other medical personnel. As everybody knows that these people are so prestigious in the society and some of us compare them with the God.

  Launching and marketing new medical objects is challenging as the consequences are critical

  These doctors and medical personnel are quite busy and therefore, it is not simple for the pharmaceutical sales representatives to interact with these personnel for presenting/ selling their products.

- **How do you think you would get a Physician to switch to your drug?**

  The biggest challenge comes with a physician who is happy with his current drug. In such a case, your first step is to make your presence felt by setting small goals and making small in roads. As you gain more knowledge about the drugs and the physician's prescribing behavior you would use your product knowledge and other tools to make the physician view your drug favorably. Then your next step is to get the physician to prescribe to one patient type, and you have a foot in the door. Follow up with the Doctor to see the results on the patient type and then you can push for other patient types.

- **You are given a territory and a list of physicians to call on. How would you organize and prioritize your call schedule?**

  Nothing beats sound field knowledge to make a strategy know your territory first.

  Know your customers and their sales potential.

  Analyze the data and figure out where your biggest potential is in terms of the 80:20 principle of (80% of your business comes from 20% of the people).

  After the A list is covered, then make your own B list and C list within a time frame that fits with the organizations sales closing.

- **What is the hierarchy of pharmaceutical marketing?**

  Refer to 4.2.4

- **What is pH?**

  Refer to 5.4

  pH of blood is 7.4

  pH of urine is 6.8 to 8.6

- **What are the different systems of your body?**

  There are 9 systems. They are as follows

      Nervous System

Sense Organ

Cardiovascular System

Respiratory System

Digestive System

Execratory System

Reproductive System

Skeletal & Muscular System

Endocrine System

- **What are the different dosage forms?**

Refer to 5.4

- **What is Pharmacokinetic?**

Pharmacokinetics, sometimes described as what the body does to a drug, refers to the movement of drug into, through, and out of the body—the time course of its absorption, bioavailability, distribution, metabolism, and excretion.

It is the study of effect of body on the drug.

- **What is Pharmacodynamic?**

Pharmacodynamics is the study of the biochemical and physiological effects of drugs on the body or on microorganisms or parasites within or on the body and the mechanisms of drug action and the relationship between drug concentration and effect.

It is the study of effect of drug on the body.

- **What is Antigen & Antibody?**

A toxin or other foreign substance which induces an immune response in the body, especially the production of antibodies is called as antigen

A blood protein produced in response to and counteracting a specific antigen is called as antibody. Antibodies combine chemically with substances which the body recognizes as alien, such as bacteria, viruses, and foreign substances in the blood.

- **What is Blood?**

The fluid that circulates in the principal vascular system of human beings and other vertebrates is known as blood. Blood in humans consist of plasma in which the red blood cells, white blood cells, and platelets are suspended.

- **What is Blood Pressure?**

It is the pressure exerted by blood on the walls of blood vessels.

When your heart beats, it pumps blood round your body to give it the energy and oxygen it needs. As the blood moves, it pushes against the sides of the blood vessels. The strength of this pushing is your blood pressure. Normal B.P. is 120/80 mmHg

High Blood Pressure (Hypertension) >140mmHg = Systolic B.P. >90mmHg = Diastolic B.P.

Low Blood Pressure (Hypotension) <90mmHg = Systolic B.P. <60mmHg = Diastolic B.P.

- **What are the components of Blood?**

Blood is a specialized body fluid. It has four main components: plasma, red blood cells, white blood cells, and platelets. Blood has many different functions including transporting oxygen and nutrients to the lungs and tissues.

- **What are Vaccines & its functions?**

A vaccine is an inactivated form of bacteria or virus that is injected into the body to simulate an actual infection. Because the injected microorganisms are 'dead,' they don't cause a person to become sick. Instead, vaccines stimulate an immune response by the body that will fight off that type of illness.

Vaccines create immunity that protects you from an infection without causing the suffering of the disease itself.

- **What is Immune System**

There are special cells in our bloodstream called **white blood cells**. They have the very important job of fighting off foreign invaders such as viruses and bacteria. These invaders are known as **antigens**. White blood cells are like the armed forces of our body. They are constantly on the lookout for antigens that have entered our body, compromising our health.

We also have a group of defensive proteins circulating in our blood that are known as **antibodies**. They float around in non-active form until triggered by an immune response, such as the detection of an antigen. When this happens, billions of additional antibodies are produced that will fight off that particular antigen. This enormous army of antibodies now joins in the attack with the white blood cells, and the germs don't stand a chance.

For example, imagine that an **influenza** virus has entered your body and has begun replicating. The white blood cells patrolling your bloodstream have spotted these antigens. They gather their troops, produce a few billion antibodies geared to fight this specific virus, and launch a massive attack.

- **How diseases occur?**

Diseases occur as a result of interaction between an agent, a host and the environment.

A disease 'agent' is defined as a substance living or non-living the excessive presence or relative lack of which may initiate the disease process in man. Examples of living agents are: bacteria, viruses, fungi etc.

Host is the organism in which diseases occur and for us man is considered as host for all practical purposes. A number of host factors such as age, sex, nutritional status etc. can affect a disease.

Environment is a set of conditions under which human beings live and can be defined as "all that which is external to individual human host living or non-living and which he is in constant interaction". This includes all of man's external surroundings such as, air, water and sanitation.

- **What are Sera?**

Blood serum (Blood - Sera extracted from an animal that has immunity to a particular disease. The serum contains antibodies to one or more specific disease antigens, and when injected into humans or other animals, it can transfer immunity to those diseases.

- **What are Antisera?**

Antiserum (plural: *antisera*) is blood serum containing polyclonal antibodies and is used to pass on passive immunity to many diseases.

- **What is Analgesic?**

An *analgesic* or painkiller is a drug used to achieve *analgesia*, relief from pain. *Analgesic* drugs act in various ways on the peripheral and central nervous systems. They can be narcotic (opium derivatives like morphine, heroin etc.) or non narcotic.

Non narcotic analgesics are also known as non steroidal anti-inflammatory drugs (NSAID). Ex: Aspirin, Ibuprofen, Diclofenac etc.

- **What is Antipyretic?**

An Antipyretic is the agent which decreases the elevated body temperature.

Ex: Paracetamol

- **What is Vitamins?**

A vitamin is an organic compound and a vital nutrient that an organism requires in limited amounts. There are 2 types of vitamins:

Water soluble Vitamin (Vit B&C)

Fat soluble Vitamin (Vit A,D,E,K)

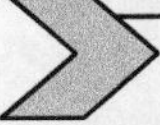

5.6 Questions for Hospital & Retail Pharmacy

- **Why do you want to join here?**

Being a graduate in Pharmacy I am very much interested to create my career in Hospital/Retail Pharmacy.

Now a days this field is growing.

- **How much hospital, Retail experience have you had?**

  Tell if you have otherwise show your eagerness by saying I am a fresher & want to build my career in this field.

- **What do you know about this field?**

  Explain clearly all the aspects of Retail Pharmacy

- **What is one of the major issues facing pharmacy today?**

  To maintain variety of drugs

- **Would relocating be a problem?**

  No, relocating is not a problem for me.

  I can manage

- **How do you handle stress?**

  By diverting my mind towards my work

- **Have you ever had a major conflict with a doctor/patient? If so, how did you handle it?**

  My 1st intention is the organization benefit & for this I can do anything.

  Thought or reaction questions and behavioral interview questions might be similar to the following:

- **How would you deal with an irate customer?**

  By providing him some extra care

- **What makes you better for this position than other candidates?**

  My ability and presence of mind.

- **Choose a topic relating to pharmacy, and we'll ask you a question about it.**

  Select the topic you prefer the most, so that you can answer the entire question asked by the interviewer.

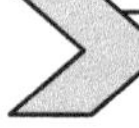

5.7 Questions for Pharmacovigilance & Clinical Data Management (CDM)

- **What is Pharmacovigilance?**

  Pharmacovigilance is the science of collecting, monitoring, researching, assessing and evaluating information from healthcare providers and patients on the adverse effects of medications, biological products, herbal and traditional medicines.

- **What are the objectives in Pharmacovigilance?**

  Understanding the concept of ADR, Medical Errors, Public Health Significance, Regulatory Interventions, ADR Monitoring schemes

- **What are the types of Pharmacovigilance?**

  There are two types of PV

  (i)   **Active PV**: Active (or proactive) safety surveillance means that active measures are taken to detect adverse events. This is managed by active follow-up after treatment and the events may be detected by asking patients directly or screening patient records. The most comprehensive method is cohort event monitoring (CEM)

  (ii) **Passive PV**: Passive surveillance means that no active measures are taken to look for adverse effects other that the encouragement of health professionals and others to report safety concerns. Reporting is dependent on the initiative and motivation of the potential reporters. This is the most common form of Pharmacovigilance. It is commonly referred to as "spontaneous" or "voluntary" reporting.

- **What to report in PV?**

  Patient Details (Name, Address, Sex, Date of Birth, Weight & Height), Patient medical history of significance, Details of Medicines (Generic or brand name, Formulation, mode of administration & Indication), Reaction Details, Date and place of report.

- **What are the Data Assessments in Pharmacovigilance?**

  Individual case report assessment, Aggregated assessment & interpretation, Signal detection, Interactions & risk factors, Serial study, Frequency and Estimation.

- **What is an Adverse Drug Event (ADE)?**

  Any untoward medical occurrence in a patient or clinical investigation subject after administering a pharmaceutical product

- **What is an Adverse Drug Reaction (ADR)?**

  An adverse drug reaction is a "response to a drug which is noxious and unintended and which occurs at doses normally used in man for prophylaxis, diagnosis, or therapy of disease or for the modification of physiologic function." There is a causal link between a drug and an adverse drug reaction. An adverse drug reaction is harm directly caused by the drug at normal doses, during normal use.

- **What is the difference between an ADE and ADR?**

  There may not be a causal relationship between a drug and an ADE, whereas, there is a causal link between a drug and an adverse drug reaction.

- **What is the minimum criterion required for a valid case?**

  (i)   An identifiable reporter

  (ii) An identifiable patient

(iii)   A suspect product

(iv)   An adverse drug event

- **What is unexpected adverse reaction and expected adverse reaction?**

  An unexpected AE is any adverse reaction not observed whether or not it has been anticipated because of the pharmacologic properties of the study agent.

  An expected AE is any adverse reaction whose nature and intensity have been previously observed and documented for the study product (e.g. in the investigator brochure, product information).

- **Process in Pharmacovigilance**

  Collect and record of AEs/ADRs

  Causality assessment and analysis of ADRS

  Collate and code in database

  Compute risk benefit and suggest regulatory action

  Communicate for safe use of drugs among stakeholders

- **What do you mean by causality?**

  Causality is the relationship between a set of factors. In Pharmacovigilance, causality is the relationship between the suspect product and the adverse drug event.

- **Causality Assessment**

  It is the evaluation of the likelihood that a medicine was the causative agent of an observed adverse reaction.

- **What is compliance?**

  The faithful adherence of the patient to the prescriber's instructions.

- **What is control group?**

  A control is the standard by which experimental observations are evaluated. In many clinical trials, one group of patients will be given an experimental drug or treatment, while the control group is given either a standard treatment for the illness or a placebo.

- **Absolute risk**

  Risk in a population of exposed persons; the probability of an event affecting members of a particular population (e.g. 1 in 1000). Absolute risk can be measured over time (incidence) or at a given time (prevalence).

- **Attributable risk**

  Attribute risk is the result of an absolute comparison between outcome frequency measurements, such as incidence.

- **Database**

  Database specifies the conditions and reservations applying to interpretations and use of the data.

- **Placebo**

  A placebo is an inactive pill, liquid, or powder that has no treatment value. In clinical trials, experimental treatments are often compared with placebos to assess the experimental treatment's effectiveness. In some studies, the participants in the control group will receive a placebo instead of an active drug or experimental treatment.

- **When do you consider an event to be serious?**

  If an event is associated with any one of the following, it is considered to be serious

  (i)   Death

  (ii) Life threatening

  (iii) Hospitalization or prolongation of hospitalization.

  (iv) Congenital anomaly

  (v)   Disability

  (vi) Medically significant

- **Name the regulatory bodies in USA, UK, Japan and India?**

  USA: United States Food and drug administration (USFDA).

  UK: European Medicines Agency (EMEA).

  Japan: Ministry of Health, Labour and Welfare (MHLW).

  India: Central Drugs Standard Control Organization (CDSCO)

- **What is Volume 9A?**

  Volume 9A brings together general guidance on the requirements, procedures, roles and activities in the field of pharmacovigilance, for both Marketing Authorisation Holders (MAH) and Competent Authorities of medicinal products for human use; it incorporates international agreements reached within the framework of the International Conference on Harmonisation (ICH).

  Volume 9A is presented in four parts:

  Part I deals with Guidelines for Marketing Authorisation Holders;

  Part II deals with Guidelines for Competent Authorities and the Agency;

  Part III provides the Guidelines for the electronic exchange of pharmacovigilance in the EU

  Part IV provides Guidelines on pharmacovigilance communication.

- **When do you consider a case to be medically confirmed?**

  A case is considered to be medically confirmed if it contains at least one event confirmed or reported by an HCP (Health Care Professional)

  Note: HCP can be a physician, nurse, pharmacist.

- **Name some data elements in ICSR (Individual Case Report)?**

  Patient demographics: Age, gender and race.

  Suspect product details: Drug, dose, dosage form, therapy dates, therapy duration and indication.

  Adverse event details: Event, event onset date, seriousness criterion, event end date and latency.

- **What should a narrative consist of?**

  A narrative should consist of precise and concise information about the source of report, patient demographics, patient's medical history, concomitant medications, suspect product details and adverse event details in an orderly manner.

- **What do you mean by MedDRA?**

  Medical Dictionary for Regulatory Activities.

- **Explain the hierarchy in MedDRA.**

  System Organ Class (SOC)

  High Level Group Term (HLGT)

  High Level Term (HLT)

  Preferred Term (PT)

  Lower Level Term (LLT)

- **What do you know about E2a, E2b and E2c guidelines?**

  E2a: E2a guidelines give standard definitions and terminology for key aspects of clinical safety reporting. It also gives guidance on mechanisms for handling expedited (rapid) reporting of adverse drug reactions in the investigational phase of drug development.

  E2b: E2b guidelines for the maintenance of clinical safety data management and information about the data elements for transmission of Individual Case Safety Reports.

  E2c: E2b guidelines for the maintenance of clinical safety data management and information about the Periodic Safety Update Reports for marketed drugs.

- **What is a Protocol?**

  A protocol is a study plan on which all clinical trials are based. The plan is carefully designed to safeguard the health of the participants as well as answer specific research questions. A protocol describes what type of people may participate in the trial; the schedule of tests, procedures, medications, dosages and the length of the study. While in a clinical trial, participants following a protocol are seen regularly by the research staff to monitor their health and to determine the safety and effectiveness of their treatment.

- **What is Clinical trial?**

  A systematic study on pharmaceutical products in human subjects (including patients and other volunteers) in order to discover or verify the effects of and/or identify any adverse reaction to investigational products, and/or to study the absorption, distribution, metabolism and excretion (ADME) of the product with the objective of ascertaining their efficacy and safety.

- **Preclinical Study in short.**

  Objective: To gather efficacy, toxicity and pharmacokinetic information of the drug in testing on non-human subjects,

  Dose: Unrestricted

  Typical number of participants: Not Applicable

- **Different Phases of clinical trials?**

  Phase 0

  Objective: Pharmacokinetics particularly oral bioavailability and half-life of the drug

  Dose: Very Small, Sub-therapeutic

  Typical number of participants: 10 People

  Notes: often skipped for phase I

  Phase I studies assess the safety of a drug. This initial phase of testing, which can take several months to complete, usually includes a small number of healthy volunteers **(20 to 100)**, who are generally paid for participating in the study. The study is designed to determine the effect of the drug or device on humans including how it is absorbed, metabolized, and excreted. This phase also investigates the side effects that occur as dosage levels are increased. About 70% of experimental drugs pass this phase of testing.

  In Phase I trials, researchers test an experimental drug or treatment in a small group of people (20-80) for the first time to evaluate its safety, determine a safe dosage range, and identify side effects.

  Phase II studies test the efficacy of a drug or device. This second phase of testing can last from several months to two years, and involves up to several hundred patients **(100-300)**. Most phase II studies are randomized trials where one group of patients receives the experimental drug, while a second "control" group receives a standard treatment or placebo. Often these studies are "blinded" which means that neither the patients nor the researchers know who has received the experimental drug. This allows investigators to provide the pharmaceutical company and the FDA with comparative information about the relative safety and effectiveness of the new drug. About one-third of experimental drugs successfully complete both Phase I and Phase II studies.

In Phase II trials, the experimental study drug or treatment is given to a larger group of people (100-300) to see if it is effective and to further evaluate its safety.

Phase III studies involve randomized and blind testing in several hundred to several thousand patients **(300-300)**. This large-scale testing, which can last several years, provides the pharmaceutical company and the FDA with a more thorough understanding of the effectiveness of the drug or device, the benefits and the range of possible adverse reactions. 70% to 90% of drugs that enter Phase III studies successfully complete this phase of testing. Once Phase III is complete, a pharmaceutical company can request FDA approval for marketing the drug.

In Phase III trials, the experimental study drug or treatment is given to large groups of people (1,000-3,000) to confirm its effectiveness, monitor side effects, compare it to commonly used treatments, and collect information that will allow the experimental drug or treatment to be used safely.

Phase IV studies, often called Post Marketing Surveillance Trials, are conducted after a drug or device has been approved for consumer sale. Pharmaceutical companies have several objectives at this stage: (1) to compare a drug with other drugs already in the market; (2) to monitor a drug's long-term effectiveness and impact on a patient's quality of life; and (3) to determine the cost-effectiveness of a drug therapy relative to other traditional and new therapies. Phase IV studies can result in a drug or device being taken off the market or restrictions of use could be placed on the product depending on the findings in the study.

In Phase IV trials, post marketing studies delineate additional information including the drug's risks, benefits, and optimal use.

- **What is Clinical Data Management (CDM)**

  Clinical Data Management (CDM) is a critical phase in **clinical** research, which leads to generation of high-quality, reliable, and statistically sound **data** from **clinical** trials. **Clinical data management** assures collection, integration and availability of **data** at appropriate quality and cost.

- **Objectives of CDM**

  CDM is a vital vehicle in Clinical Trials to ensure:

  The Integrity & quality of data being transferred from trial subjects to a database system

  That trial database is complete and accurate, and a true representation of what took place in trial

  That trial database is sufficiently clean to support statistical analysis, and its subsequent presentation and interpretation

- **Importance of CDM**

  CDM has evolved from a mere data entry process to a much diverse process today

  It provides data and database in a usable format in a timely manner

  It ensures clean data and a ready to lock database

- **What is database lock?**

  The database lock for a study is done to ensure no manipulation of study data during the final analysis

- **What is SAE Reconciliation?**

  Serious Adverse Event (SAE) data reconciliation is the comparison of key safety data variables between Clinical Data Management System (CDMS) and Sponsor PV. Reconciliation is performed to ensure that events residing in both systems are consistent.

- **Describe SDTM?**

  CDISC's Study Data Tabulation Model (SDTM) has been developed to standardize what is submitted to the FDA.

- **What is CRF?**

  A **case report form** (or **CRF**) is a paper or electronic questionnaire specifically used in clinical trial research. The **case report form** is the tool used by the sponsor of the clinical trial to collect data from each participating patient.

- **What is annotated CRF?**

  Annotated CRF is a CRF (Case report form) in which variable names are written next to the spaces provided to the investigator. Annotated CRF serves as a link between the raw data and the questions on the CRF. It is a valuable tool for the programmers and statisticians.

- **What is CRT?**

  Case Report Tabulation, whenever a pharmaceutical company is submitting an NDA, company has to send the CRT's to the FDA.

- **Formulary**

  A listing of medicinal drugs with their composition, uses, method of administration, available dose, dosage forms, side effects etc.

- **Allopathy**

  Allopathy is a non-traditional, western scientific therapy, usually using synthesized ingredients, but may also contain a purified active ingredient extracted from a plant or other natural source, usually in opposition to the disease.

- **Homeopathy**

  According to homeopathy an illness is treated with a medicine which could produce similar symptoms in a healthy person. In Homeopathy treatment, the active ingredients are given in highly diluted form to avoid toxicity.

- **Biological Products**

  Biological products are medical products prepared from biological material of human, animal or microbiologic origin

- **Efficacy**

  Efficacy is the ability of a drug to produce the intended effect as determined by scientific methods, for example in pre-clinical research conditions.

- **Side effect**

  Any unintended effect of a Pharmaceutical product occurring at normal dosage and is related to the pharmacological properties of the drug.

- **Pharmacology**

  Study of uses, effects and modes of action of drugs

- **Pharmacoepidemiology**

  Study of the use and effects of drugs in large populations

- **Essential Medicines**

  Essential medicines are those that satisfy the priority health care needs of the population. They are selected with due regard to public health relevance, evidence on efficacy and safety, and comparative cost effectiveness.

- **Rational Drug Use**

  An ideal of therapeutic practice in which drugs are prescribed and used in exact accordance with the best understanding of their appropriateness for the indication and the particular patient, and of their benefit, harm effectiveness and risk.

- **Misuse**

  This refers to situations where the medicines I intentionally and inappropriately used not in accordance with the authorized PI or the directions for use on the medicine label.

- **Drug Abuse**

  This corresponds to the persistent or sporadic, intentional excessive use of a medicine, which is accompanied by harmful physical or psychological effects.

- **Full form of PV Terms**

ADE	Adverse Drug Event
ADRS	Adverse Drug Reactions
ART	Antiretroviral Therapy
ARV	Antiretroviral
ATC	Anatomic Therapeutic Chemical
BCPNN	Bayesian Confidence Propagating Neural Network
CEM	Cohort Event Monitoring
CIOMS	Council for International Organization of Medical Sciences
DD (WHO)	Drug Dictionary
ESTRI	Electronic Standards for the Transfer of Regulatory Information
FDA	Food and Drug Administration (USA)
HIPAA	Health Insurance Portability and Accountability Act
IBD	International Birth Date
ICD	International Classification of Diseases
ICH	International Conference on Harmonization of Technical Requirements For Registration of Pharmaceuticals for Human Use
ICSR	Individual Case Report
IMAI	Integrated Management of Adolescent and adult illness
IMMP	Intensive Medicines Monitoring Programme (The New Zealand)
ISOP	International Society of Pharmacovigilance
MedDRA	Medical Dictionary for Drug Regulatory Activities
OI	Opportunistic Infection
PEM	Prescription Event Monitoring
PSUR	Periodic Safety Update Report
PvC	Pharmacovigilance Centre
SAE	Serious Adverse Event
SOC	System Organ Class
SOP	Standard Operating Procedure
SSAR	Suspected Serious Adverse Reaction
SUSAR	Suspected Unexpected Serious Adverse Reaction
UMC	The Uppsala Monitoring Centre
VigiBase	WHO database of individual case safety (ADR) reports (ICSR)

VigiFlow	Spontaneous reporting data entry and analytical tool
VigiMine	Data mining tool available as part of VigiSearch
VigiSearch	Search tool for searching the VigiBase database
WHO-ART	World Health Organization Adverse Reactions Terminology
WHO	World Health Organization

- **Few other Full forms**

ANDA	Abbreviated New Drug Application
API	Active Pharmaceutical Ingredients
CDSCO	Central Drugs Standard Control Organization
CGMP	Current Good Manufacturing Practices
COPP	Certificates of Pharmaceutical Products
CPSC	Consumer Product Safety Commission
CQA	Corporate Quality Assurance
CRO	Contract Research Organization
DCGI	Drug Control General (India)
DSP	Dry Sterilization Process
EDQM	European Directorate of Quality Medicines
EUGMP	European Union Good Manufacturing Practice
FEFO	First expired first out
FICCI	Federation of Indian Chambers of Commerce & Industry
FIFO	First in first out
GAMP	Good Automated Manufacturing Practice
GCP	Good Clinical Practice
GDP	Good Distribution Practice
GLP	Good Laboratory Practice
GMP	Good Manufacturing Practice
ICMR	Indian Council of Medical Research
ICH	International Conference on Harmonization
IDMA	Indian Drug Manufacturing Association
INDA	Investigational New Drug Application
IPA	Indian Pharmaceutical Association
IPQA	In-Process Quality Assurance
ISPE	International Society for Pharmaceutical Engineering
IVRI	Indian Veterinary Research Institute
MCC	Medicines Control Council (in South Africa)
NIPER	National Institute of Pharmaceutical Education & Research

OTC	Over the Counter
OPPI	Organization of Pharmaceutical Producers of India
PQLI	Product Quality Life Cycle Implementation
PQS	Pharmaceutical Quality System
QBD	Quality by Design
QMS	Quality Management System
SAL	Sterility Assurance Levels
SOP	Standard Operating Procedure
SPDS	Society for Pharmaceutical Dissolution Science
TGA	Therapeutic Goods Administration (in Australia)
TRP	Tamper Resistant Packaging
UK MHRA	United Kingdom's Medicines and Health products Regulatory Agency
UNESCO	*United Nations Educational, Scientific and Cultural Organization*
USFDA	United States Food and Drug Administration
WHO	World Health Organization

- **Government & Regulatory Bodies**

International	International Conference on Harmonisation (ICH)
	United Nations Health Care Organization (UNHCO)
	World Health Organization (WHO)
	World Trade Organization (WTO)
Argentina	Ministry of Health
	National Administration of Drugs, Food & Medical Technology (ANMAT)
Armenia	Drug and Medical Technology Centre
	Ministry of Health
Australia	Australia's Department of Health and Aged Care
	Therapeutic Goods Administration (TGA)
Austria	Bundesministerium für Gesundhe
Bahrain	Ministry of Health
Bangladesh	Ministry of Health
Belgium	Federal Public Service (FPS) Health, Food Chain Safety and Environment

Belize	Ministry of Health
Bolivia	Ministry of Health and Sports
Botswana	Ministry of Health
Brazil	Ministry of Health
	National Health Surveillance Agency (Anvisa)
Brunei	Ministry of Health
Bulgaria	Bulgarian Drug Agency (BDA)
Canada	Health Canada
Chile	Ministry of Health
China	State Food and Drug Administration (SFDA)
Colombia	Ministry of Health
	National Institute of Food and Drug Monitoring (INVIMA)
Costa Rica	Ministry of Health
Croatia	Ministry of Health and Social Welfare
Cuba	Ministry of Public Health
Czech Republic	State Institute for Drug Control
Denmark	Danish Medicines Agency
Ecuador	Ministry of Public Health
Egypt	Ministry of Health and Population
El Salvador	Ministry of Health
Estonia	State Agency of Medicines
Europe	EU Legislation - Eudralex
	European Directorate for the Quality of Medicines and Healthcare (EDQM)
	European Medicines Agency (EMEA)
	Heads of Medicines Agencies (HMA)
Fiji	Ministry of Health
Finland	Finnish Medicines Agency
France	Agence Française de Sécurité Sanitaire des Produits de Santé
	Ministry of Health
Georgia	Ministry of Labour, Health and Social Affairs of Georgia
Germany	Federal Institute for Drugs and Medical Devices (BfArM)
	Ministry of Health
	Paul-Ehrlich-Instituts in Langen (PEI)

Greece	National Organization for Medicines (EOF)
Guam	Department of Public Health and Social Services
Guatemala	Ministry of Health and Welfare
Guyana	Ministry of Health
Hong Kong	Department of Health: Pharmaceutical Services
Hungary	National Institute for Pharmacy
Iceland	Icelandic Medicines Agency
	Ministry of Health & Social Security
India	Central Drug Standard Control Organization (CDSCO)
	Government of India Directory of Health and Family Welfare
	Indian Council of Medical Research (ICMR)
	Ministry of Health and Family Welfare
Indonesia	Ministry of Health
Ireland	Department of Health and Children
	Irish Medicines Board
Israel	Ministry of Health
Italy	Italian Pharmaceutical Agency
	Ministry of Health
Japan	Ministry of Health and Welfare
	National Institute of Infectious Diseases
	National Institute of Health Sciences
Jamaica	Ministry of Health
Jordan	Ministry of Health
Kenya	Ministry of Health
Latvia	State Agency of Medicines
Lebanon	Ministry of Public Health
Lithuania	State Medicines Control Agency
Luxembourg	Ministry of Health
Malaysia	National Pharmaceutical Control Bureau
Maldives	Ministry of Health and Family
Malta	Medicines Authority
	Ministry of Health
Mauritius	Ministry of Health and Quality of Life

Mexico	Ministry of Health
Morocco	Ministry of Health
Namibia	Ministry of Health and Social Services
Nepal	Ministry of Health and Population
Netherlands	Medicines Evaluation Board
New Zealand	Medsafe - Medicines and Medical Devices Safety Authority
	New Zealand Ministry of Health
	PHARMAC
Nicaragua	Ministry of Health
Nigeria	National Agency for Food and Drug Administration and Control (NAFDAC)
Norway	Ministry of Health and Care Services
	Norwegian Medicines Agency
Pakistan	Drug Control Organisation, Ministry of Health
Palestine	Ministry of Health
Panama	Ministry of Health
Papua New Guinea	Department of Health
Paraguay	Ministry of Health
Peru	Ministry of Health
Phillipines	Department of Health
	Philippine Council for Health Research and Development (PCHRD)
Poland	Ministry of Health & Social Welfare
Portugal	The National Institute of Pharmacy and Medicines (Infarmed)
Romania	Ministry of Health
	National Medicines Agency (ANM)
Russia	Association of International Pharmaceutical Manufacturers
	Ministry of Health and Social Development
	Public Health Institute
Saudi Arabia	Ministry of Health
Senegal	Ministry of Health and Prevention
Serbia	Medicines and Medical Devices Agency (ALIMS)
	Ministry of Health

Singapore	Health Sciences Authority (HSA)
	Ministry of Health
Slovak Republic	Ministry of Health
	State Institute for Drug Control (SIDC)
Slovenia	Ministry of Health Agency for Medicinal Products
Sri Lanka	Ministry of Healthcare and Nutrition
South Africa	Department of Health
	Medicines Control Council (MCC)
South Korea	Food and Drug Administration
Spain	Medicines and Health Products Agency (AEMPS)
	Ministry of Health
Sweden	Medical Products Agency (MPA)
Switzerland	Swiss Agency for Therapeutic Products
Taiwain	Department of Health
Tanzania	Ministry of Health and Social Welfare
Thailand	Ministry of Public Health
Trinidad and Tobago	Ministry of Public Health
Tunisia	Ministry of Public Health
	Office of Pharmacy and Medicine
Turkey	Ministry of Health
Uganda	National Council for Science and Technology (UNCST)
Ukraine	Ministry of Health
United Arab Emirates	Ministry of Health
UK	Association of the British Pharmaceutical Industry (ABPI)
	Department of Health
	Medicines and Healthcare Products Regulatory Agency (MHRA)
	National Health Service (NHS)
	National Institute for Biological Standards and Control (NIBSC)
	Prescription Services NHS
Uruguary	Ministry of Public Health

USA	Centers for Disease Control and Prevention
	Department of Health and Human Services (DHHS)
	FedWorld - US Government Information
	The Food and Drug Administration (FDA)
	National Center for Complementary and Alternative Medicine (NCCAM)
	National Institutes of Health (NIH)
	National Library of Medicine
	National Science Foundation
	Office of Disease Prevention
Venezuela	Ministry of Public Health
Vietnam	Ministry of Health
Yemen	Ministry of Public Health and Population

CHAPTER 6

Few Employers

- ## Clinical Research

  Quintiles: It is the only fully integrated biopharmaceutical services company offering clinical, commercial, consulting and capital solutions worldwide. Its network of 23,000 engaged professionals in 60 countries around the globe works with an unwavering commitment to patients, safety and ethics — ensuring a higher level of healthcare for people. For its biopharmaceutical customers, it helps them navigate risk and seize opportunities in an environment where change is constant.

  (quintiles.taleo.net/careersection)

  Parexel: It has supported the Bio-Tech and Pharmaceutical industries in helping the development of new drugs and treatments on a global basis. As a leading global biopharmaceutical service provider, they supply knowledge-based contract research, medical communications and consulting services across a broad range of therapeutic areas to the worldwide pharmaceutical, biotechnology and medical device industries. They have helped over 800 clients to develop and launch some of the most important drugs and devices of our time-helping people live better and healthier lives everywhere in the world. Headquartered near Boston, Massachusetts, Parexel operates in more than 50 countries around the world.

  (https://www.parexel.com)

  quantity and quality.

- ## Pharmacist

  The National Rural Health Mission (NRHM): It was launched in April 2005. The NRHM focused especially on 18 states, with poor infrastructure and low public health indicators, namely the eight Empowered Action Group (EAG) states - (Bihar, Jharkhand, Madhya Pradesh, Chhattisgarh, Uttar Pradesh, Uttaranchal, Odisha and Rajasthan), the eight North Eastern States (Assam, Arunachal Pradesh, Manipur, Mizoram, Meghalaya, Nagaland, Sikkim, Tripura) and two other states, namely, Himachal Pradesh and Jammu & Kashmir

- **Hospitals**
  - Apollo Hospitals
  - Batra Hospitals
  - Wockhardt Hospital
  - Fortis Hospital
  - Amri Hospital
  - Escort Hospital
  - Tata Memorial Hospital
  - L V Prasad Eye Hospital
  - All India Institutes of Medical Sciences

- **Emergency Medical Technician (Ambulance)**
  - Ziqitza Health Care Limited
  - Web Site: www.zhl.org.in

- **Health Advice Officer**

  HMRI

  Health Management & Research Institute is an NGO having Partnership with **Govt. of Maharashtra & Piramal Health care**. Health Management and Research Institute is a registered non-profit organization based in Hyderabad, Andhra Pradesh. **HMRI** is supported by Piramal Foundation and works towards making healthcare accessible, affordable and available to all segments of the population, especially those most vulnerable

  Contact Details

  HMRI,

  3rd Floor, Pune Chest Hopital,

  Near Old Sangvi Phata

  Anudh, Pune – 411 027

- **Medical Coding**

  GeBBS Healthcare Solutions Pvt. Ltd.

  4th floor, building no.5, Mindspace,

  Thane-Belapur road, Airoli, Opp Airoli railway station,

  Mumbai – 400 708

  Omega Healthcare Management Services

  Bangalore Office Address:

  Omega Healthcare Management Services Pvt. Ltd.,

  33, NAL Wind Tunnel Road, Bangalore – 560 017

  Phone: +91 80 4155 7333

Chennai Office Address:
Omega Healthcare Management Services Pvt. Ltd.,
9th Floor, Tower -2, RMZ Millennia Business Park,
No.143, Dr MGR Road, Kandanchavadi,
Chennai - 600 096
Phone: +91 44 49070101

Epi Source India Pvt. Ltd.
18, Satyanarayana Avenue, Boat club Road, R.A. Puram
Chennai, Tamil nadu - 600 020
Fixed Phone: 044-42031560
Mobile: 09884041315
Email Id: contact@epi-source.com

- **Pharmacovigilance**

Cognizant Technology Solutions
13th, Kensington SEZ
Hiranandani Business Park
Powai, Mumbai - 400 076
India
Ph: +91- 22 – 4422 8000
Fax: +91-22-4422800

Accenture Services Pvt. Ltd.
Green Boulevard,
2d floor, Tower B & C, B9A, Block B,
Sector 62, Noida, Uttar Pradesh - 201301
Phone: 0120 476 4000
Divyasree Technopark,
SEZ, SY NO 36/2 Kundalahalli Village,
K R Puram Hobli, White Field
Brookefield, Bangalore 080-4077 0100

Mind Tree Ltd.
Mindtree Ltd. Global Village,
RVCE Post, Mysore Road, RVCE Main Rd,
Mailasandra, Bangalore, Karnataka 560 059
Phone: 080 67 064000
Rajiv Gandhi Infotech & Biotech Park,
Plot No.37 Phase 1. MIDC, Hinjewadi Pune - 411 057.
Maharashtra, INDIA
Phone: +91 20 3915 6000

Norwich Clinical Services Pvt. Ltd.
No.147/F, Arc Mansion,
8th Main Road, 3rd Block,
Koramangala, Bangalore – 560 034
Phone: (080) 42772400

Tata Consultancy Services
Vidyasagar Building, Off Western Express Highway,
Near Saibaba Temple, Raheja Township
Western Express Hwy, Malad East,
Mumbai, 022 6779 8585
Standard Design Factory II, Unit 61
Santacruz Electronic Export Processing Zone,
Andheri East, Mumbai

- ## Medical Transcriptionist & Quality Analyst

  Drugmol Informatics: It has been a one-stop solution center based in Bhopal with a captive client in all fields which take care of the clients present globally. (career@drugmol.com)

- ## Patient Care Advisor

  Indigene: It is scientific and competitive intelligence services lend actionable insights to clients to support their strategic decision making. It provides scientific, clinical, and competitive insights to help align the business development, licensing, clinical development, and marketing activities of its clients to current and future market needs. (www.indegene.com/careers)

- ## Pharma Manufacturing

  Alkem Laboratories Ltd.
  C-6/1,C-6/2, C-17/7, MIDC Industrial Estate, Taloja, Taluka Panvel
  Raigad, Navi Mumbai- 410 208

  Allele Life Science (P) Ltd
  C-59 , Sector-10 , Noida - UP 201301, www.allelelifesciences.org
  E.Mail- allelelifescience@gmail.com,
  Phone: +91-0120- 4271978 / 3994522, 2442676, 3053625,
  Mobile: 9891179928, 9818185261

  AstraZeneca India Pvt. Ltd.
  Bellary Road, Hebbal, Bangalore - 560 024

  Bharat Serums & Vaccines Ltd.
  R&D Centre, DIL Complex
  Near Tatwagyan Vidyapeeth, Ghodbhunder Road
  Thane (West) 400 610, 16th Floor, Hoechst House, Nariman Point,
  Mumbai – 21

Blue Cross Laboratories Ltd.
Peninsula Chambers,
P.O. Box 16360,Lower Parel, Mumbai - 400 013

Caplin Point Laboratories Ltd
Narbavi, No.-3, Lakshmanan Street, T.Nagar, Chennai - 600 017

Cipla Ltd
M-61 to M-63, Verna Industrial Estate, Verna Salcette, Goa- 403 722
Near Teesta River,, Kumrek, Rangpo, Gangtok - 737 132
Sikkim,India, www.cipla.com

Dr. Reddy's Laboratories Ltd.
Ward-F,Block-4, TS No.-8/2,& 8/4
Adavipolam Industrial Area, Yanam - 533 464

Dr. Reddy's Laboratories Ltd.
Innovation Plaza, Survey Nos. 42,45,46&54
Bachupalli, Qutubullapur, RR Dist - 500 072, A.P

Excel Life Sciences
B-155, 2nd Floor, Sector- 63, Noida - 201 301, U.P.

Fresenius Kabi
Fresenius Kabi Oncology Ltd., 19, HPSIDC, Industrial area
Baddi - 173 205, Solan, Himachal Pradesh

Glenmark Generics Ltd.
B/2, Mahalaxmi Chambers., 22 Bhulabhai Desai Road
Mumbai 400026
Plot No.- S-7, Colvale Industrial Estate
Bardez., Goa - 403 513

Healthy Pharma
Mr.Neshith Shah, Director
Healthy Life Pharma Pvt. Ltd, 401, Richa, B-29, New Link Road,
Andheri (w), Mumbai - 400 053
Tel: 022 - 32459914 , Fax: 022 - 67415973
Email: info@healthypharma.com, www.healthylifepharma.com

Ipca Laboratories Ltd.
Plot No.-65&99, Danudyog Industrial Estate
Vapi, Silvasa-396230
48, Kandivli Industrial Estate, Kandivli (West), Mumbai - 400 067

Khandelwal Laboratories Pvt. Ltd.
B-1, Wagle Industrial Estate
Thane - 400 604

Matrix Laboratories Ltd.
F-4 & F-12, MIDC, Malegaon, Sinnar
Nashik - 422 113

Max Neeman International
Vipra Datta, Sr. Manager HR
Max House, 1st Floor, 1, Dr. Jha Marg, Okhla-III
New Delhi - 110 020

Medo Pharm
Medo House, 25, Puliyar II Main Road,
Trustpuram, Chennai - 600 024

Micro Advanced Research Centre
Corporate R&D Centre, (A Unit of Micro Labs Ltd)
58/3, Singasandra Post, Hosur Road, Kudulu
Bangalore - 560 068

Natco Pharma Limited
Nalco House, Road No.2, Banjara Hills, Hyderabad-500033
info@natcopharma.co.in

Ranbaxy Laboratories Ltd.
Industrial Area-3, Dewas - 455 001, M.P.

Sandoz Private Ltd.
MIDC Plot No.-8-A/2, 8-B, T.T.C. Ind. Area
Kalwe Block, Village Dighe, Navi Mumbai - 400 708

Sanmour Pharma
99/1/2, Shreenidhi, Near Mahindra Showroom
Ghodbunder Road, Owala, Thane (W) - 400 607

Siddhayu Ayurvedic Research Foundation Pvt. Ltd.
(A Group company of Baidyanath)
Ph: +91 712 2702391 / 6644923
www.siddhayu.com, www.baidyanath.co.in

SK Health Care Formulations Pvt. Ltd.
Manager Operations, 8-58/5, I.D.A. Bollaram Road
Batchupally (V), R.R.Dist, Hyderabad - 500 072

Sterling Biotech Ltd.
Jambusar State Highway, Village Massar - 391 421
Padra,Vadodara, Gujrat

Sun Pharma

Acme Plaza, Andheri Kurla Road, Andheri (East), Mumbai - 400 059

Plot No.-754 Setipool, Ranipool, East Sikkim - 737 135

Syngene International Pvt. Ltd.

Biocon Park, Plot No. 2 & 3, Bommasandra IV Phase

Bangalore - 560 099, careers@syngeneintl.com

Wanbury Ltd.

A-15, MIDC Industrial Area

Patalganga, Raigad - 410 220, Maharastra

Watson Pharm

Plot No.-A3 to A6, Phase I-A

Verna Industrial Estate, Verna, Salcette, Goa - 403 722

Wockhardt Ltd.

Kunjhal, Barotiwala, Nalagarh, Solan

Himachal Pradesh - 174103

Wockhardt Tower, Bandra Kurla Complex

Bandra (East), Mumbai - 400 051

List of few Pharmaceutical Industries

A

Abbott Laboratories

Actavis

Add-Life Pharma Ltd

Ahlcon Parenterals (India) Ltd

Ajanta Pharma

Albert David Ltd

Alchemist Ltd

Alembic Ltd

Alexion Pharmaceuticals

Alkem Laboratories

Allergan Pharma

Alpha Laboratories Ltd

Altana Pharma AG

Ambalal Sarabhai Enterprises Ltd

Amgen Pharma

Amico Laboratories

Amrutanjan Health Care Ltd

Anavex Life Sciences

Ankur Drugs & Pharma Ltd

Apotex Inc.

Arvind Remedies Ltd

AstraZeneca Pharma

Auro Laboratories Ltd

Aurobindo Pharma Ltd

Aventis Pharma Ltd

Axcan Pharma

B

Bacil Pharma Ltd

Bafna Pharmaceuticals Ltd

Bajaj Healthcare Limited

Bal Pharma Ltd

Baxter International

Bayer Schering Pharma

BDH Industries Ltd

Beryl Drugs Ltd

Beximco Pharma

Beximco Pharmaceuticals Ltd

Bharat Biotech Ltd

Bharat Serums & Vaccines Ltd

Biocon Limited

Biofil Pharmaceuticals Ltd

Bionovo

Bliss GVS Pharma Ltd

Brabourne Enterprises Ltd

Brawn Pharmaceuticals Ltd

C

C S C Pharmaceuticals

Cadila Healthcare Ltd

Caplin Point Laboratories Ltd

Celestial Labs Ltd

Celogen Pharma

Centaur

Centenial Surgical Suture Ltd

Cipla Ltd

Colinz Laboratories Ltd

Consolidated Pharmaceuticals Ltd

Coral Laboratories Ltd

Core Healthcare Ltd

D

DIL Ltd

Diffusion Pharmaceuticals

Dishman Pharmaceuticals Ltd

Divi'S Laboratories Ltd

Dr. Reddy's Laboratories Limited

E

Ego Pharmaceuticals

Élan Corporation

Elder Pharmaceuticals

Eli Lilly and Company

Endo Pharmaceuticals

Everest Organics Ltd

F

F. Hoffmann–La Roche Ltd

Ferring Pharmaceuticals

Flemingo Pharma

Forest Laboratories

Fresenius Kabi Oncology Ltd

Fulford (India) Ltd

G

Galapagos NV

Galderma Laboratories

Genentech

Genzyme Pharmaceuticals

Getz Pharma

Gennex Laboratories Ltd

Gilead Sciences

GlaxoSmithKline

Glenmark Pharmaceuticals

Godavari Drugs Ltd

Granules India Ltd

Group Pharmaceutical

Gufic Biosciences Ltd

Gulf Pharmaceutical

Gujarat Inject (Kerala) Ltd

Gujarat Terce Laboratories Ltd

H

Harleystreet Pharmaceuticals Ltd

Help Remedies

Helsinn

Hester Biosciences Ltd

Hetero Drugs

Hexal Australia

Hikma Pharmaceuticals

Hindustan Bio Sciences Ltd

Hiran Orgochem Ltd

Hoffmann–La Roche

Hospira Pharmaceuticals

I

IMULAN BioTherapeutics, LLC

Incepta Pharmaceuticals

Indoco Remedies Ltd

Ind-Swift Laboratories Ltd

Inwinex Pharmaceuticals Ltd

Intas Biopharmaceuticals

Intercytex

Interphil Laboratories

Ipca Laboratories Ltd

Ishita Drugs & Inds. Ltd

J

Jagsonpal Pharmaceuticals Ltd

JB Chemicals & Pharmaceuticals Ltd

Janssen Pharmaceuticals

Jenburkt Pharmaceuticals Ltd

Johnson & Johnson

JK Pharmachem Ltd

Jubilant Organosys Ltd

Jupiter Bioscience Ltd

K

Kappac Pharma Ltd

KDL Biotech Ltd

Kerala Ayurveda Ltd

Kilitch Drugs (India) Ltd

Kontest Pharmaceuticals

Kopran Ltd

Krebs Biochemicals & Inds. Ltd

L

Lactose (India) Ltd

Lark Laboratories Ltd

Lincoln Pharmaceuticals Ltd

Lupin Limited

Lyka Labs Ltd

M

Mangalam Drugs & Organics Ltd

MannKind Corporation

Marksans Pharma Ltd

Matrix Laboratories Limited

MDI

Medi-Caps Ltd

Medo Pharm

Merck Ltd

Morepen Laboratories Ltd

Millennium Pharmaceuticals

Mylan

N

Naprod Life Sciences Pvt Ltd

Natco Pharma Ltd

Natural Capsules Ltd

Nectar Lifesciences Ltd

Neuland Laboratories Ltd

Nova Bay Pharmaceuticals

Novartis

Novo Nordisk

O

Octa Pharma

Omkar Pharmachem Ltd

Orchid Pharmaceuticals Ltd

P

Panacea Biotech Ltd

Panchsheel Organics Ltd

Panjon Ltd

Par Pharmaceutical

Parenteral Drugs (India) Ltd

Pfizer Ltd

Phaarmasia Ltd

Pharmaids Pharmaceuticals Ltd

PI Drugs & Pharmaceuticals Ltd

Piramal Healthcare Ltd

Plethico Pharmaceuticals Ltd

Principal Pharmaceuticals Ltd

Purdue Pharma

R

Ranbaxy Laboratories

Respa Pharmaceuticals

Rubra Medicaments Ltd

Rubicon Research

S

Salix Pharmaceuticals

Samrat Pharmachem Ltd

Saamya Biotech (India) Ltd

Sandu Pharmaceuticals Ltd

Sanjivani Paranteral Ltd

Sanofi-Aventis

Serum Institute of India

Sigma Pharmaceuticals

Sino Pharm Group

SMS Pharmaceuticals Ltd

Solvay Group

Square Pharmaceuticals

Sterling Biotech Ltd

Strides Arcolab Ltd

Sun Pharmaceutical Limited

Supriya Pharmaceuticals Ltd

Surya Pharmaceutical Ltd

Suven Life Sciences Ltd

Sword & Shield Pharma Ltd

T

Teva Pharmaceuticals

Themis Medicare Ltd

Theon Pharmaceuticals

Torrent Pharmaceuticals

Transchem Ltd

Triochem Products Ltd

Troika Pharmaceuticals

TTK Healthcare Ltd

Twilight Litaka Pharma Ltd

U

UCB

Unichem Laboratories Ltd

Unjha Formulations Ltd

United Laboratories

V

Valeant Pharmaceuticals

Vardhaman Laboratories Ltd

V-Ensure

Vapi Care Limited

Venus Remedies Ltd

Vertex Pharmaceuticals

W

Wallace Pharmaceuticals

Wanbury Ltd

Watson Pharma

Welcure Pharmaceuticals Ltd

Wincare

Wockhardt Limited

Wyeth Ltd

Z

Zandu Pharmaceutical Works Ltd

Zenith Health Care Ltd

Zenotech Laboratories Ltd

Zentiva

Zuventus Healthcare

Zydus Cadilla

www.ingramcontent.com/pod-product-compliance
Lightning Source LLC
LaVergne TN
LVHW080848240726
843527LV00052B/267